Earth Mama's
Spiritual Guide to
Weight Loss

Be relaxed, in control and calm

STEPHANIE ROSE BIRD

Green Magic

Green Magic
5 Stathe Cottages
Stathe
Somerset TA7 0JL
England

www.greenmagicpublishing.com

Designed and typeset by K.DESIGN.
www.k-design.org.uk

ISBN 9780995547841

GREEN MAGIC

Dedication

To the women in my family, who have maintained, shifted, transformed and held steady in their selves and weight, Aunt Rose, Aunt Joan, Aunt Edith, my Mom and Mother-in-Law, Iris. Your spirited journeys shaped this book, and are inspirational. I dedicate this book to you.

Contents

Preface

I am what many people would call an Earth Mama. As an avid butterfly and wildflower gardener, herbalist, natural product designer, landscape painter, botanical arts instructor, companion to four animals, wife and mother of four children, I amply fit the profile.

Bringing my children into the world, nursing them and watching them grow are the pride and joy of my life. The problem is I have been growing and expanding exponentially with each child, averaging a 60-pound weight gain per child. As a young woman, I found it relatively painless to lose the 180 pounds gained with the first three children, but my late in life baby was an altogether different story.

If you thought it was impossible for any woman to wear a few more hats, think again. In addition to my mothering roles, I am also a healer and shaman. These blessings help me cope with the more challenging aspects of life. When I used to have trouble casting off those extra 60 pounds I turned to the realm of magic, nature and goddess-lore to find support that doctors and nutritionists did not supply.

Sadly, I found there wasn't a single book focused on weight-loss using alternative spirituality and complementary medicine.

Therefore, I took it upon myself to research recipes, treatments and programs that hold promise. I noticed that aromatherapy, using my collection of essential oils, provided relief from anxious feelings during my strict diet. Essential oils elevated my mood and amused me during the low points when I might have indulged in over-eating. The essential oils were added to my bath and since I often have baths while burning incense, I found that combining the two, inspired deep relaxation and focus on achieving my goals. I knew that flower essences offer gentle but effective treatment for a variety of personality issues and psychological challenges so I began exploring their possibilities with great results.

One of the more surprising discoveries made along the way was that hypnotism is a very effective way of supporting a diet plan. I first learned of this by watching a case study on Dateline NBC. I was so impressed with the massive amount of weight the subject lost that I began to search for a local hypnotist with a good reputation. The first place I searched was through our local hospital fitness program and fortunately, they had a hypnotist who led groups in smoking cessation and weight-loss programs. I went through a screening process with her and set up a series of appointments.

You must understand that, when I went to see her, I was a basket case in terms of my diet. This was shameful to me as an herbalist but a reality nonetheless. I would sit at my computer most days munching and quickly finishing bags of cookies, chips or ultra-rich candy bars. I knew that anxiety and boredom led to the eating but I could not stop myself, it seemed fun – that is, until I'd get up and have a look at myself in the mirror. I was shocked and humiliated because I was huge, not just a little overweight.

I had spent my youth actively involved in dance as a performer. When I stopped performing I began teaching aerobics and jazzercise. Gradually my family and professional life superseded gym activities. In my 30's I could barely look at myself, yet day after day I'd continue the same old eating pattern. I had kept some of my limberness from stretching as a dancer and my body seemed surprisingly sound for quite a while but eventually it too began to cave in. My back hurt terribly and so did my knees. In short, I was a mess. I knew that chances were I'd never be as active as I once was since I had changed lifestyles from an active dancer to an artist, writer and mom but there had to be some light at the end of the tunnel I had dug.

My first visit to the hypnotist was nothing short of magical. We talked and I spoke of the psychological issues that I thought led to my over-eating. She listened patiently but judging from the battery of allergy tests I had run previously, and from my eating patterns, she decided rather quickly that I was a carbohydrate addict. She felt that there was a strong biological component to overeating rather than the psychological element that so many of us focus on. She suggested several books featuring a high protein low carbohydrate regime created by a couple of authors she trusted. As a do-it-yourself type, I listened but I knew I wasn't one to stick to a certain dieting scheme, especially if it seemed to be a popular fad diet. I wrote down the books, we chatted a bit longer and then we began the hypnotism session.

She had me lay back in a comfortably overstuffed leather chair and then tilted the chair back so that my feet were elevated. She began playing taped music that was very relaxing. She then began her gentle coaxing and guidance. Before I knew it, I was 14 years old, coming of age in a very small bikini, submerged in the ocean in Cape May, New Jersey. The sun was beaming overhead warming the blue-tinged salt water. I was underwater yet I could breathe freely. This seemed to go on infinitely though in reality it was only about 20 minutes. The message she planted in my mind was "I am relaxed, I am in control, and I am calm." "Fat cannot protect you; strong and lean, is fit and powerful." I find myself calling upon these words as a daily mantra and affirmation.

I knew that although the diet books she recommended weren't appealing, it would behoove me to research the implications and cures for carbohydrate and sugar addiction.

Being that I love anthropology, particularly the study of ancient cultures, I gravitated towards "NeanderThin" and "The Paleolithic Diet" (Paleo is the popular name). These diets are high in protein low in carbohydrates and prohibit simple carbs like soda, candy and chips. Since I am very involved in earth-based spirituality, I was drawn to the author's approach of eating natural, unprocessed foods the way our earliest ancestors did. I've always loved nuts and this diet encourages consumption of all types of raw nuts, nut milks, berries, vegetables, fruits and of course meat, which is somewhat problematic for me, as I don't eat red meat. I decided that I could only eat what my conscience allowed, which excludes red meat. Still, with fish, fowl, nuts, vegetables and certain herbs I was able to receive ample protein. Within 10 days of seeing the therapist (and this is not to say it will happen for everyone) I had lost 12 pounds.

Soon enough though I grew tired of food groups being left arbitrarily out of my diet such as legumes and dairy. I was also bothered by eating fish and fowl. Today, I eat mainly fruits, vegetables, nuts and legumes, as a vegetarian. I am happier, feel more humane and seem to be healthier eating a plant-based diet. I have been diagnosed with IBS (irritable bowel syndrome) so I limit wheat, avoid gluten and limit my intake of milk-based dairy products, while not excluding them entirely. This simple eating regimen, food journaling and controlling my portions has facilitated a sense of being grounded in the earth, which has led to weight-loss.

Now, when you have 90 pounds to lose, you know that you are in it for the long haul. I decided to get help around the house in the ways I know best. I spiritually cleansed my altar and added some special flowers and foods as offerings to my ancestral spirits. I planted a few of my own vegetables and herbs amongst my flowers, so that I could tend to them and watch them grow. Perhaps the most special places in my home though were the kitchen and bath.

My kitchen became like a holy shrine to my weight-loss. I discarded unhealthy foods and began replacing them with special herbal teas, seeds, nuts, berries, veggies and legumes. I meticulously cleaned and sanitized the cutting board, sharpened the kitchen knives and put fresh flowers on the windowsill to offer gentle support. The stove and refrigerator were cleansed (inside and out) with a combination of lemon and orange essential oils, baking soda and white vinegar. I posted eating guides concerning the glycemic index on the fridge and cabinets.

No domestic goddess, I did my best to keep things neatly arranged, not a small task with such a lively household. Finally, I called up the goddesses of health Xel Chel and Hestia to keep my kitchen energy positive and reinforcing. I looked above my sink at my collection of dried corn and thanked the Corn Mothers, goddesses of fertility and harvest. The goddesses remind me on a daily basis that food is a sacred symbol of fertility, the fruit of a great harvest. Food is something to be shared, savored and enjoyed but never something to be greedily devoured to excess without giving thanks.

Of course, eating live whole foods is not all spiritual; they require energy in preparation and acquisition. I dug up my old health-conscious magazines and cookbooks. My juicer was cleaned and I invested in a high-powered blender for fruity protein drinks. I returned to my health-food haunts. I dusted off my bike and began riding instead of driving to get the food, sometimes when there was only a few things to buy I walked, carrying the groceries in a backpack. I increased the intensity of my household cleaning, not content to limit this great energy to the kitchen. I began to garden more and spend more time outside with my children. All of this not only kept me busy but it burned calories and left less time to sit around ruminating over impending failures or emotional injuries from the past. It seemed like my days of freedom had returned, moreover I was winning the battle over food – it didn't consume me, I consumed it with purpose and joy.

The bathroom became a shrine of sorts as well. With the ample water and tea consumption, I was constantly in and out of the bathroom. I wanted it kept aromatic and appealing so I began cleaning it too with tea tree oil and lemongrass. Lighting incense is now a daily activity, especially the lovely Nag Champa from Thailand. Nag Champa helped me suspend judgments I simply contemplated my progress. I took numerous baths, sometimes several times a day because water is such a powerful place of grounding and centering. I created my own sea salt blends in honor of Yemoya-Ologun, Nigerian orisha (spirits) of the sea. This made each bath a relaxing, sensory treat, as my Yemoya-Ologun blend includes eucalyptus, lemon verbena, peppermint, bay leaf, lavender, baking soda, Dead Sea salt and plenty of the muscle relaxant Epsom Salt. A few seashells, stones, botanical soaps and natural products had transformed my bath from a place for doing business to an aromatic oasis in my home.

The bathroom was quickly transforming into a sacred personal space for thanking my body.

Following are a few personal affirmations that you might consider adopting:

- I thank my body for being the perfect temple of my soul
- I thank my body for being capable and strong
- I thank my body for its willingness to learn new habits
- I thank my body for letting part of itself go
- I thank my body for welcoming and supporting change
- I beg my body, please allow this transformation to be complete

I found these affirmations to be perfectly suitable accompaniments to soaping up my hands, rinsing my body, applying scented lotions and oils or simply as I'd recline and relax in a bubble bath.

Now that I've shared a little of my personal journey with you I invite you to take the journey of connection to the Earth Mama. The journey is towards wholeness, completion, health and self-realization. Come along; bring your sensible weight-loss program, read **Earth Mama's Spiritual Guide to Weight-loss**: *How Earth Rituals, Goddess Invocations, Incantations, Affirmations and Natural Remedies Enhance Any Weight-loss Plan."* and work steadily on meeting your personal goals.

Part I

Wisdom of the Sages
Indigenous and Earth-based
Knowledge

CHAPTER 1

Dawn in the Dreamtime

Australia c. 1993: Journey to the Dreamtime

I was probably at my fittest, most healthy state, I have been as an adult, when I spent the year in Australia. My daughter was 18 months old. I had recently broken my arm very badly. Noticing how I carried myself, catering to the arm, my adopted clan on Elcho Island, also called Galiwin'ku by the Yolngu people, named me the English equivalent of Broken Stick. Yes, it had been a challenging journey to get there. Apparently, it showed.

Back to the fitness part though. I went to Australia to live among the Aborigines because I was drawn to their paintings. All the paintings called to me, from the x-ray styled work of the Top-End, near Elcho Island, where I stayed the longest, to the so-called dot-styled dreamings of the central Australian desert region, or even the broad, amorphous shapes of the Western Kimberly area. The paintings called to me. Called me away from my job as an art professor. Called me to raise enough money to bring my entire family to Australia.

Of course, to understand the paintings, I would also need to understand the people who painted them. After all, it was also photographs of these earthy Black people that drew me in – calling me to action. Bare-legged women and often barefoot as a people, I was drawn to the way the Aboriginal Australians of the Outback seemed to live so closely to nature. From what I could see, they didn't just live closely to nature, they lived as one with her.

I am from a rural area of New Jersey. For a while, my family lived very close to nature too, due to the circumstances of our house being built on a meager budget and us not having running water for about a year. Having lived in Philadelphia, San Diego's La Jolla and the Chicago area, I craved the time I could once again live closely to nature.

Traveling to the geographic center of the compelling and inspirational paintings led me to not only live 'out bush' with the people of various language groups and clans, what we would mistakenly call tribes but what are actually clans; also to gain an inner understanding of Aboriginal Australian and Torres Strait Islander's ancient way of life.

With no television, or in some cases indoor-plumbing, electricity and scanty grocers, if any, I quickly adapted to an ancient way of living. I dispensed with wearing shoes, in most cases, and instead tread directly on the Earth Mama. Fire became the center of our lives. Around the fire was the place for gathering to socialize, to cook, eat and listen to stories. Water was the source of inspiration and sustenance. In the desert the air was hot and dry, whereas, the Top-End tropics, experienced both an extremely wet season and an arid hot and dry one.

I had some baby weight on me. Typically, I gain at least 60 pounds during pregnancy, as I said. This is a testament to my food addiction, as much as it is to my desire to nurture new life.

I found that without exerting the slightest bit of effort, without concentration or deprivation, the weight I was carrying after giving birth magically melted away. Now, you may be wondering if I bought a magic wand with me. Indeed, I did not. Instead, I involved myself deeply with the rhythms of the Aboriginal way of life, in the communities where I lived. I was lucky to go to every major area accept Southern and Western Australia.

Storytelling was important to filling our day with wonder and joy. Building and maintaining fires, that took physical exertion, that I suppose burned calories. Going to the sea to gather crustaceans and mollusks in our dilly bags to eat – that too expended energy. We would go out into the bush, or out bush, as the Australian's call it, to gather bush tucker – otherwise, what we would call wild foods through scavenging. Even going to the single grocer on Elcho Island at the time, meant a good long walk and then carrying the groceries back. Natural weightlifting, you might as well say.

To be honest though, food was for sustenance and not feeding addictions, such as my addiction to sugar. Expensive to buy, arduous to hunt and gather, food and its consumption, what with the fire-building and all, well, it required work.

Chocolate, my stalwart friend, was quickly replaced by the desire to hear simple clap stick music, the didgeridoo and most of all, having the opportunity to dance in a ritual or participate in a ceremony. Plus, chocolate was damned expensive. At $2.50 for a simple Hersey's candy bar, all the way back in the early 1990's.

You get it by now. In my experiences living in remote outback Aboriginal Australian communities, run by Elder Councils, I learned by example to be a healthier person, fit in mind, body and spirit.

The take away from my experience, living with a people considered having the longest direct history to our earliest days, a lineage approximately 60,000 years of unbroken history as humans, was that dieting doesn't enable you to enjoy the level of mental and physical fitness I enjoyed Down Under. To achieve that level of inner and outer satisfaction requires something else entirely. Your soul must be fed a good and healthy diet of art, music, storytelling, dancing, ritual and ceremony. Moving naturally, within the verdant arms of Earth Mama, that is what did the trick.

Women's Business and Women's Law

There was another concept that impacted how I saw life – women's business and men's business. As a woman, I was not privy to men's business. Being much as it sounds, men's business and women's business or law, contains a huge reservoir of the law as set by the creator ancestors during the dreamtime. The dreamtime is not fixed in a long off distant epoch, rather it ranges from the conception of the world, right into the present day.

One thing I cherished about women's business was the Elder Crones who held the key to this knowledge. By crone, I am referring to elders, generally beyond child-bearing age, who have also acquired deep knowledge about life, over time. The women, gifted with the unique set of knowledge called women's business, were their own kind of leaders, mentors and healers.

We are all going to grow old, if luck is on our side. What better gift could we be given than to be revered for our knowledge of ourselves, our environment and community? What I saw, and admired, in the women entrusted with Women's Law was women who had a deep knowledge of wild foods, ancient ceremony and ritual that included intricate storytelling, song, dance and visual art, such as painting and crafts. The melding of that broad-based knowledge that brought together ancient earth-based spirituality with the arts, practical knowledge and history, yielded a powerful ability to heal.

In a nutshell, this unique set of knowledge, I so admire in Aboriginal Australian Women's Business, is something you can access in your own way through this book. Some of you will become more familiar with various gods, goddesses, supernatural beings, and spirits for the first time. Then you will take that new-found knowledge and put it to use. Learning from their stories, trials, tribulations and triumphs. Others of you will already be familiar with the figures and concepts discussed within these pages. Your task will be to renew and deepen your connection to them, as you apply these lessons to your weight-loss journey.

Lessons of the Djanggawul Sisters

The Djanggawul Sisters and their brother, are dreamtime creation ancestors, important especially to the Yolngu people, of which I am an adopted member. I am sharing their story in this first chapter because it is a cautionary tale. The sisters simply had to touch the earth in a certain way and a new natural feature or formation would be created. These are powerful beings.

Naturally, as creation ancestors, much of the Djanggawul Sister's time was spent either conceiving, being pregnant or giving birth. The sisters, Bildjiwuraroju is the oldest, whereas, Miralaidj, is the younger one, are fertility Mothers of northeastern Arnhemland — the place I previously describe as my home away from home. The sisters came across the seas, traveling in their canoe. They bought

21

powerful symbolic objects with them, which revolve around fertility, such as an nganmara (a symbolic uterus).

The Djanggawul protected and sheltered women and children, with their knowledge and sacred objects, such as dilly bags and a special pandanus mat. Pandanus is used widely in Arnhemland as a weaving tool and grows naturally there. These women created some of the most important rituals to the dua moiety.

THE DILLY BAG

A dilly bag is a handmade bag, usually about 1½ feet long and about 8" wide, made from locally harvested materials and colored with natural dyes. They have a long history in the Top End of Australia (Northern Australia) in a place traditionally called Arnhemland. The bags feature prominently in creation stories of the dreamtime. Dilly bags are still used for harvesting, gathering, fishing, hunting, rituals and ceremonies.

When the Djanggawul sisters went to Marabai to rest, they hung up their dilly bags and baskets filled with sacred objects. Away collecting mangrove shells, their brother and his friends, stole the sacred baskets. Within the baskets were sacred creation songs and powerful rituals. The sisters were frightened to hear the men singing their sacred songs.

The sisters lost the baskets but maintained their knowledge within themselves. The lesson we can all take away from the Djanggawul Sisters is that we are all pregnant with magical creative possibilities. Pregnancy and fertility can symbolize personal potentiality. We can also birth things from our minds, into creation, including a new, healthier self. It is important to stay focused on all that is sacred and important to you and remain vigilantly attendant to it so it is not lost.

CRAFTING A DJANGGAWUL SISTER BAG

SUPPLY LIST

Kraft paper lunch bag

Drawing Materials such as: Fine point Sharpies
(fine point markers) Crayons or Cray-pas (oil pastels),
Colored Pencils or Chalk Pastels.

Glitter Glue

Scissors

1. Decorate a simple, brown craft paper lunch bag. Have fun with this, using glitter glue, markers and cray-pas.

2. Cut white unlined (printer) paper, into ½″ × 4″ strips, like the paper strip found in a fortune cookie.

3. Write a sentence describing the parts of yourself you feel you have lost, due to being overweight or obese. Limit yourself to ten words.
    For example: I am no longer as physically active as
                  I use to be.

4. Now on the flip side of the paper, write the solution.
    For example: I will walk twice a week for 15 minutes.

5. Create 12 of these pieces of paper – one for each month of the year.

6. Tri-fold them and put them in the decorated bag.

7. Pick your frequency; I suggest once a week if you have less than 20 pounds to lose and once a month if you have over 50 pounds to shed.

8. Read both sides of the sheet of paper.

9. Take action to change your habits according to the wisdom that has been revealed.

TIPS

- Once you tackle the issue represented on the sheet of paper dispose of it by burning it. Return the ashes to Earth Mama.
- Make another sheet to replace the previous one.
- Continue this process for a year (or longer, if like me, when I started this process, you have more than 75 pounds to lose).

Gaia's Gifts

Gaia is the European representative of the Great Mother. She is one of the Great Goddesses of the world. It is my hope that you will find your soul well-fed by Gaia's gifts--that you will internalize the affirmation given and try some of the suggestions for prayers, altars, potions, rituals and ceremonies. The goal is for you to gain control over food addiction, if that is your struggle. At the very least, you will hopefully gain control of your types of consumption. You will have aid as you struggle through the difficulties of transformation and change. Ultimately, you will be able to take a fresh look at yourself and embrace the new you that comes out of this work.

The Eden Within

I know we can't all just take off for parts of the world generally unknown. We can however do what is in our power to find this sort of Eden I describe within ourselves. This book is about getting past calorie counting and deprivation. It is about celebration of nature, and the gods and goddesses that formed it as well as the spirits that bring it to life. Through these stories, lessons, rituals, prayers, invocations, incantations and affirmations, you will naturally find the inner peace that allows your body to shed or release, unwanted, unnecessary heaviness. The largeness of nature and all its creation stories, ancestor beings, healing medicines and gifts, will hopefully fill you up in a way that food cannot.

Take a moment. Look at how you are living right now. Chances are, if you are heavier than you'd like to be, you are also quite sedentary. Now, think back to your ancestors. Imagine what they had to do every single day to survive and sustain their families. Quite a different picture, don't you think?

My African-descended ancestors worked as enslaved people on tobacco plantations and as servants. Most of us, sitting in our air-conditioning, on a comfy couch, couldn't begin to understand how taxing being an enslaved person might have been. Taxing, not just to the mind but grueling on the body and spirit. I have to take a deep breath and do an open-mouthed sigh, just thinking about it.

More recently, think about your parent's lives. You will probably see in your mind's eye people who worked very hard but also who took the time to cook and make sure you were taken care of.

In my case, as I vision quest back into the 60's and 70's, I see that my people didn't suffer from obesity and its ills nearly as much as they do today. With no computers and less choice on television, folks got out, on their feet and were active. When I think back on those times, the striking features I remember are slow-cooked and home-cooked meals, often with vegetables and fruits harvested from our side garden. I remember singing in gospel choirs and that equally fed my soul. Then too, there was lots and lots of dancing.

So, just looking at personal history, which could stand for the story of many with slight adaptations, you find first deep ancestry, intimately connected to movement and the earth. Closer ancestors who worked hard physically and sustained themselves expressively through art like singing and dancing. Even as I think back on my parents, a mother I considered fat (who never in her wildest dreams came close to my heaviest weight), I see that my people filled up on a different kind of food. Hand-made, slow-cooked, locally harvested food, digested along with friends and family, rather than in front of multiple screens, as in smart phones and HDTV.

Dream Keepers: Lessons of Shaman

A very small, though important part of my ancestry is Native American. One of the more fascinating aspects of Native American culture in relation to this conversation about slimming down, is the notion of shamanism and within the area of Shamanism lives the concept of shape shifting.

Shaman are not limited to the world so many of us are stuck in. They have lower world, middle world and upper world. They can travel the astral planes to the different worlds that make up our existence.

Admirable and useful to you on your personal journey towards weight-loss is the shaman's way of dreaming the world, calling up an unimagined world into being. Secondly, though there is no hierarchy here, is the shaman's ability to vision quest. Rather than explaining away about vision quests, how about I take you through one here and now?

Goddess Spirituality and a Vision Quest

Several years ago, okay, let's be more realistic, over a decade ago, I was a board member of a Goddess-oriented Women's Spirituality group. One of our most memorable activities was an exercise to find our power animals, animal spirit allies or animal totem.

I wasn't quite sure what to expect, since I had already learned through dreaming I was closely aligned with bear energy and could shape shift into a she-bear. I was so closely attuned to bear that I became her during lucid dreaming.

Well, lo and behold, I did not find bear energy during my vision quest. Instead I found that I was a furry rat. Don't laugh. I felt dismayed but it made sense, since I was also born in the year of the Rat. I will get more into the attributes of the rat and other animals, which you might find during your vision quest, shortly.

I am making this one of your first activities because whether you call it your animal totem, animal spirit ally or power animal, you want to identify this aspect, aligned with yourself. You will need your animal to guide, inspire, mentor, protect and enlighten you on this challenging journey to shed unwanted weight.

There are many ways to go about finding your animal. Some people do it as simply as meditating on an animal card deck. When I was with the women in my Goddess Spirituality group, this is how we did it.

Finding Your Power Animal

1. Find a safe place, where you will be uninterrupted by loud sounds or other intrusions, which would create stress or tension. I suggest a remote outdoor location, if possible.
2. Lie down on your back and close your eyes.
3. Have your arms relaxed and on the ground, lifted out and away from the sides of your body.
4. Turn your palms upward, so the backs of your hands touch the earth.
5. Let your palm be opened and relaxed. (This is a receptive posture)
6. Relax your face muscles; open your mouth slightly.
7. With your eyes closed, imagine your eyes almost crossing, as each tries to focus, at the same time, on the bridge of your nose.
8. Now, concentrate on your breathing and nothing else. Try breathing in to the count of 6 or 8 and out on the same count. Get lost in your breathing, while letting your other thoughts fall away. Let everything else disappear by the wayside.
9. Feel your body cradle into Earth Mama's lap. Relax and only focus on your breath.
10. Next, imagine your mind is a chalk board. Take an eraser and wipe it clean. Every time a new thought arises, notice it and then erase it from the board with an eraser.
11. Go back to your breathing. Stay there until you are completely and totally relaxed.
12. Now, ask your animal to reveal itself to you. Observe, but do not judge. Ask yourself to notice, how does it move, what does it see, how does it smell, what does it look like?
13. Congratulations! You have met your power animal.

Animal Wisdom

As you make your way on this journey, over the next few weeks, months or even years, I want you to listen to your animal. Your animal is with you and will always be with you, even when you don't think you need it or see it.

Now that I've piqued your interest and you've done your personal vision quest, I want to share a few of the highlights of some of the major iconic Animal Totems. This is just a glimpse into the possibilities that your animal holds.

Animal Totem Sampler

Armadillo	shielded, chivalrous, protective, strong, sensitive
Antelope	sensitive, communicative, fast, psychic
Badger	solitary, storytelling, earth-wise, fierceness
Bat	strength, stamina, perception, transitions, facility
Beaver	crafty, dreamer, skillful, strategic, building/planning
Bison	strength, grounded, abundance, sacred, manifesting, action, adaptable
Cougar	stealthy, self-possessed, decisive, assertive
Coyote	cooperative, wise, trickster, primal
Deer	virginal, clairvoyant, innocent, perceptive
Dolphin	passionate, creative, endurance, perceptive
Elephant	strength, power, wisdom, sensuality, loyalty

Elk	power, strength, regal, cooperative, social
Fox	shape shifter, feminine, magical, invisible, adaptable, energetic
Giraffe	seer-visionary, friendly, family-orientated, strategic
Goat	prophetic, grounded, stable, flexible
Horse	clairvoyant, persuasive, free, adventurous, sensitive
Lion	cooperative, leader, protective, stealthy, intuitive, emblem of the sun
Moose	shape shifter, contradictory, longevity, sexual, adaptable, primal-feminine
Mouse	detail-orientated, fastidious, adaptable, earthy, grounded
Opossum	trickster, covert, strategic, far-sighted, prepared
Otter	loving, fun, social, playful, whimsical
Panther/Jaguar	mysterious, regenerative, awakening, fierce, valiant, graceful, wise
Rabbit or Hare	fertile, sensitive, artistic, susceptible, clever, fast, trickster
Raccoon	hidden, masked, concealed, changeable, curious
Ram	starter, tenacious, sacrifice, energetic
Rhinoceros	idealistic, sensitive, inherent, wisdom
Seal	artistic, imagination, survivor, dreamer, emotional

Skunk	sensual, adaptable, repellant, attractive, defensive
Squirrel	judicious, active, busy, prepared, planner
Tiger	adventurous, powerful, self-possessed, sensual, ferocious
Weasel	consumptive, graceful, secretive, aggressive, trickster
Whale	creative, perceptive, knowing, resurrection, musical/song/breath
Wolf	frugal, communicative, ritualistic, discerning, protective

---

BASTET

Egyptian cat goddess Bastet, controls birth, healing, magic, fertility and pleasure, among other parts of your life, thus you should reflect on her when considering personal transformation. She is often pictured with a cat's head and a woman's body. Bastet is watchful and protective. She protects the body from harm and ushers in smooth birthing. Her special charge includes women and healers. Bastet's sacred animal is the domestic cat.

Bird Totems

Being in touch with Father Sky and Mother Earth, people with bird totems, for better and in some cases, for the worse, can travel two distinct and different realms. Bird people are spiritual and typically powerful by nature. Here is a sampling of bird totems you might envision in your vision quest:

Blue Jay	mimics, fearless, survivor, diligent
Cardinal	spirituality, renewal, change, benevolence
Crow	potentiality, watchfulness, vigilance, magical, intelligent
Crane	longevity, justice, enlightenment, hope
Eagle	healing, shape shifting, nobility, divinity, ambition
Hawk	fearless, healer, visionary/artistic, spiritual
Hummingbird	adaptability/flexibility, tenacity, joyful, adept
Magpie	metaphysical/occultist, intelligence, knowledgeable
Owl	prophetic, magical, feminine, clairvoyant, visionary
Peacock	watchful, rising-energy, wisdom, visionary
Pelican	lightness, giving, magical, powerful
Raven	shape shifter, occultist, prophesy, magical
Stork	birthing/midwifery, dedicated, lucky, mysterious
Swan	inner and outer beauty, self-possessed, emotional, strong
Vulture	renewal, growth, change, purification, cleansing

Reptiles and Amphibians

In the corpus of shape shifting and totemic animals, seldom does such a rich history of folklore and mythology, as well as connection to gods, goddesses and spirits exist like that for reptiles and amphibians. As you read this book you will encounter a large amount of deities and spirits connected to this group, to deepen your understanding of your ability to transform.

Alligator and Crocodile	birth, death, maternity, wisdom, guardianship, mystical
Frog	metamorphosis, abundance, fertility, emotional, self-possessed, magical
Lizard	intuitive, sensitive, subtle, dreamer, detachment
Turtle	gatekeeper, sensual/sexual, longevity, primal, feminine, grounded

---

SNAKE

Snake is heavily associated with deity around the world. Snakes are extremely important to Goddess and Earth-based Spirituality. They represent the life cycles, particularly birth and death, regeneration, renewal and change, transformation, thus they are very important to your work within this book.

Researching Your Totem

Now is the time for you to make your own study of your totem, whether it is an animal, reptile, amphibian or bird. Make a list for yourself following my example here. Looking cross-culturally here is what I've found out about my animals, the rat and the bear.

Rat Attributes

Shielded

Resourceful

Easy Going

Driven

Fertile

Strong

Ambitious

Flexible

Invisible

Driven

Prophetic

Prosperous

Smart

Peaceful

Bear Attributes

Versatile

Maternal

Protective

Leader

Confident

Empathetic

Empathic

Assertive

Strong

Aggressive

Patient

Hedonist

Critical

Grounded

Psychic

Protective

Leader

Domestic

Changing Woman: Estsantlehi (es-tan-AHT-lu-hee)

You are going to go through personal transformation, employing your power animal as well as gods, goddesses and other spiritual beings as you journey. As you change mentally and physically, shifting your shape, it is good to reflect on the goddess of changes,

34

Changing Woman, also called Estsantlehi by the Navaho.

Let's not kid ourselves, slimming down takes time. Estsantlehi is the goddess of time and the changing seasons. Since you are devoting weeks, months or maybe even years to your weight-loss journey, what better goddess to inspire you?

Estsantlehi was born from a union of Father Sky and Mother Earth (Native American). She is also the Sun's wife thus she lives in the West. Their home is made of four beautiful and powerful natural substances:

- White Shell on the eastern side
- Turquoise makes up the south side
- Yellow abalone on the west
- Black jet to the north

Once the Sun and Estsantheli's children, Monster Slayer and Child of the Water, set out on their own, Estsantlehi felt the empty nest and was lonely. Brushing magical dust from between her breasts, she saw one side release flour and the other side disperse cornmeal. Making a paste with these two ingredients, she created two sets of men and two sets of women. These are the ancestors of the four Navaho clans.

You need this powerful creation goddess on your side now. Changing Woman symbolizes creativity, innovation and evolution. Possessing great strength and foresight, she is a visionary who can see herself as a maiden or crone instantaneously. Look at her as you evolve, grow spiritually as your body changes. She will remind you that life is an ever-moving circle of which you are an important part.

Affirmation

Recite the following Earth Prayer out loud as you affirm your belief
in your transformation:

O you who dwell in the house made of the dawn,
In the house made of the evening twilight . . .
Where the dark mist curtains the doorway,
The path to which is on the rainbow . . .
I have made your sacrifice.
I have prepared a smoke for you.
My feet restore for me.
My limbs restore for me.
My body restore for me.
My mind restore for me.
My voice restore for me.

Today, take away your spell from me.
Away from me you have taken it.
Far Off from me you have taken it.

Happily I recover.
Happily my interior becomes cool.
Happily my eyes regain their power.
Happily my head becomes cool.
Happily my limbs regain their power.
Happily I hear again.
Happily for me the spell is taken off.

Happily I walk.
Impervious to pain, I walk.

Feeling light within, I walk . . .

In beauty I walk.

With beauty before me, I walk.

With beauty behind me, I walk.

With beauty below me, I walk.

With beauty all around me, I walk.

It is finished in beauty.

It is finished in beauty.

It is finished in beauty

Navaho Chant

HORZHO NAASHA (Walking in Beauty)

The beauty way path informs us that beauty exists all around and within us, like light beaming through a rainbow. The rainbow attests to the existence of the divine. Horzho translates to "natural order." Natural order, as encapsulated by horzho, encompasses temporal time, the cardinal directions, and seasonal cycles, as connected back to the four directions.

Four Corn-Pollen Footsteps with the Cardinal Directions

East	childhood	sunrise, spring, morality
South	youngster	afternoon, summer, learning
West	parenthood	sunset, autumn, family
North	grand-parenting	midnight, winter, reverence for the self and nature
Center	hearth and home, spiritual love for the family	

Going through painful and challenging changes may be in order, to achieve your weight-loss goals. Once you go through this transformation, you are restoring the natural order within. You are then able to love others and yourself, fully and completely, considering carefully the four corn-pollen footsteps of the cardinal directions. Now you can move forward, walking in the beauty way.

CHAPTER 2

Apothecary of the Gods, Goddesses and Lwa

O our Father, the Sky, hear us
and make us strong.
O our Mother the Earth, hear us
and give us support.
O Spirit of the East,
send us your Wisdom.
O Spirit of the South,
may we tread your path of life.
O Spirit of the West,
may we always be ready for the long journey.
O Spirit of the North, purify us
with your cleansing winds.

Sioux Prayer

Walkabout

In the previous chapter, I spoke about going *out bush*. The outback is one thing – rather remote, keeping its distance in more ways than one from Australia's cities. *Out bush* or going to outstations, takes you even further afield.

My family and I stayed at an outstation on Australia's Top End in Arnhemland's tiny community called Mapuru. We also traveled by 4-wheel drive, to other outstations in Arnhemland going as far as Millingimbi and Raminginning, even flying to get to the more remote of them in tiny planes.

I came to find that 4-wheel drives and six-seat airplanes were a part of the new walkabout. As effective as those modes of transportation are, especially for getting to funerals, rituals and ceremonies, I prefer the good old fashioned walkabout on foot. Walking, as we know, is good for the mind, body and spirit.

Two of my most enjoyable experiences in Australia, came about walking in the bush. I was led by one of my adoptive Aboriginal relatives. She taught me about how to recognize tasty bush tucker and how to eat bush foods, also known as wild-crafting and wild foods.

Another time, I went out into the bush with a group of women and children, who were basket makers. They showed me how to use simple digging sticks, a tool that the creation ancestors' use in dreamtime, to dig up roots used as natural dyes. That one field trip on foot led me to become a papermaker and soap-maker using natural dyes from plants for both.

There is a great deal of nourishment in bush tucker or wild-crafted foods gathered from the wild open spaces of the bush or elsewhere. Much of that knowledge for how to identify these foods has fallen by the wayside with time. In this chapter, which asks you to engage with Goddesses, Gods and lwa from diverse cultures in our world, focuses in on herbs and wild foods that can be used in your efforts to get trimmer. First stop – Haiti.

LWA

Lwa are not gods or goddesses. They are found in the Vodou Pantheon and in some of the African belief systems of the Bizango, Congo, Ibo and Nago people. Some lwa traveled from Africa to the Caribbean, finding a new home in places like Haiti. Lwa (spelled loa in French) are like spirits. They are sometimes considered angels or saints; most were once alive, so they are more of a supernatural being. Some are syncretized with saints. They are called variously:

- Les Saintes (the saints, since they are syncretized with Catholic Saints)
- Les Anges or Zanj (the angels)
- Les Racines (ancestral spirits or roots)
- Les Mysteres (the mysteries)
- Les Invisibles (the invisible ones)

They communicate through ritual and possession, often mounting people.

The Hidden Knowledge of Gran Bwa

Gran Bwa, is a noted figure, a lwa from the Vodou pantheon. Gran Bwa, wild man of the forest, holds the keys to native plant's wisdom. A cross between a man and a tree, this celebrated lwa is owner of the considerable power of forest plants. Flowers, leaves, roots and even fallen branches are pleasing to this lwa and can be offered to him. I am beginning this chapter with Gran Bwa because

41

he holds the key to sacred botanical knowledge of wild spaces, thus he should be honored when you begin your pursuit of discerning wild medicines to use during your transformation.

Before going into this any further, you need to equip yourself with practical knowledge about herbs in terms of how to gather and use their different parts, including the leaves, berries, flowers, bark and roots. Once you have grown, gathered and harvested your herbs, you can be on your way to using them in your weight-loss journey towards good health.

Tribute to Corn Mother Selu

Even before you learn about harvesting herbs, it is important to invoke the Corn Mothers. They are a diverse group of creation and fertility goddesses honored by various Native American clans.

Selu, the Cherokee goddess, whose name literally means corn is the goddess we will be working with. She is the goddess of fertility who invites us to appreciate the Earth Mother's bountiful harvest and to utilize its sacred abundance in sustaining healing medicines.

Selu Invocation

Lay out a nice, brightly colored place mat or runner on your eating table, befitting a goddess.

Shuck some corn and put it at the center of the table.

Say: *Selu, I honor you.*

Next, pour some blue corn meal in a turquoise or blue pottery bowl.

Say: *Selu bless my harvested herbs. Let them be fruitful in my weight-loss journey.*

Blessed Be to the Corn Mothers!

Finally, lay your herbs out on this consecrated table, dedicated to Selu before you begin to process them.

Gathering and Drying Herbs

If you can't grow your own herbs or gather them from the wild you will need to go to a local farmer's market in season or utilize dry herbs. Here are the types of questions you should ask before proceeding:

- Are the herbs ethically harvested? (Be careful about barks and roots, some are over harvested.
- Are the herbs organically grown? This is the safest method for personal care products and herbs to be consumed.
- Are the prices fair, without excessive markups? Do some research and price comparisons.
- Are the herbs usually in stock, available without delays?
- Is the source convenient and practical for you?
- Is a knowledgeable person available to answer your questions?
- Start out with a local shop if possible but as you become comfortable with creating your own brews branch out into wholesale, buying herbs in bulk saves big bucks!

TIPS FOR URBAN DWELLERS

- Look for freshness (bright color, no mold or mildew, strong scent) and expiration dates on herbs.
- Grow your favorite herbs in pots on the window sill, patio, and terrace or even inside.
- Visit your local farmers market or drive outside the city to support roadside farm stands.

Gathering and Drying Herbs

If you are fortunate enough to have enough space to grow your own herbs, fruits and vegetables the following suggestions are for you.

- When gathering Mama Earth's gifts, approach plants with respect, thank them for sharing their medicines with you before harvesting.

Harvesting Leaves

Look for leaves of a consistent green color without brown or yellow spots. Harvest mid-morning, after the dew has evaporated. Gather leaves before plant begins to flower. For plants such as basil or oregano, with long growing seasons, pinch back tops to prevent flowering. (Flowering takes energy away from the main body of the plant). Keep herbs separated by type; tie the stems loosely with twine or hemp string, together in a bundle. Until you are very familiar with all the herbs, it is best to label the bundles and date them as well. Hang them up to dry immediately after harvesting to prevent mildew or deterioration.

Hang herb bundles, stem-up in an area with good circulation away from direct sunlight. The ideal temperature for the first 24 hours is 90 degrees, followed by 75–80 degrees the rest of the time. Most herbal bundles will dry between 2–3 weeks. Petals and leaves should feel light, crisp and paper-like. If there are small buds or tiny leaves which may fall off during the drying time create a roomy muslin bag to encase flowers and leaves; tie loosely with twine or hemp string at the stems. This is particularly important with seed dropping plants such as fennel or sunflowers. When herbs are completely dry, store the whole leaf and stem away from direct sunlight in dark glass or stainless steel airtight containers.

Harvesting Flowers

Select healthy flowers in the early afternoon during dry weather conditions. Flowers are extremely delicate. Take extra care not to bruise the petals, refrain from touching them, cut from the stem and allow flowers to drop into a basket. Dry smaller more delicate flowers such as lavender and chamomile whole; hang upside down, tied with twine over a muslin cloth or large bowl or wrap loosely with muslin to retain dried buds.

Use fresh flowers whenever possible. You may also freeze them in an ice cube tray filled with spring water.

Harvesting Seeds

Collect seeds on a warm dry day. Seeds need to dry in a warm airy environment. Make provisions to catch the quickly drying seeds by placing a bowl or box underneath the hanging plants.

Harvesting Bark

Bark peels easiest on damp days. Choose a young tree or bush: if possible one that has already been pruned, cut, or taken down naturally by wind or stormy conditions, to prevent damage or even death to the plant. Stripping too much bark from a tree will kill it. A thoughtful approach to Mother Nature's gifts is essential. Bark may harbor insects or moss, so wash it first and allow to dry flat on waxed paper in a location that is well-ventilated and away from direct sun light.

Harvesting Roots

Roots are ready for collecting after autumn harvest. Dig up roots after their plant has begun to wither and die down. Extract the whole root while trying not to bruise it. Like bark, roots need to be cleaned before dried, they also require ethical harvesting. Cut roots into small sections and dry in an oven set between 120 to 140 degrees. Turn and check regularly. Roots should feel light and airy like saw dust when fully dried. For marshmallow root, peel away the top layer of skin before drying in this manner.

Harvesting Berries

Use the same procedure as for bark, but remember berries and fruits take a long time to dry, about twice as long, as leaves. You will know when they are fully dry because they will become very light, wrinkled and reduced in size by nearly half. Turn frequently and check for leaking juices. Replace paper below them often to prevent growth of bacteria or mold.

Storage

Since the flavors and volatile oils of herbs mix readily store herbs separately. Label and date sterile (tinted glass bottles or stainless steel) containers and keep in a cool dark place. The final quality of your herbs depends on how well they are stored and prepared.

Herbal Medicine Extraction Techniques

Decoctions – are made by extracting the medicines from roots, bark or berries by simmering in a covered pan of water over medium-low heat for 30 minutes to 5 hours depending on toughness of herb.

Infusions – are either water-based or oil-based. Water-based infusions are teas also called *tisanes, potions* or *brews* made by extracting the volatile oils in herbs by pouring boiling distilled water over the herb, and keeping covered for 30 minutes to 1 hour. Tougher herbs may be infused by heating in water for a longer time on a very low temperature on the stove, while tightly covered.

Oil-based infusions – extract the volatile oils from herbs by putting herbal materials into a sterilized container, filling the jar to the top with loosely packed dried herbs, and then pouring preferred oil such as: olive oil, sunflower oil, almond oil or safflower oil over the plants. Cover tightly, keep away from direct sunlight and give the jar a whirl every day for 4–6 weeks (depending on desired strength).

Tinctures – are the extraction of medicinal qualities of herbs made by using 100 proof alcohol such as vodka, grain alcohol, rum or ethanol. The concentrations of volatile oils are greater in tinctures than through infusion or decoction. A sterilized jar with a cork or other tight fitting top is filled to the top of the jar with loosely packed herbal material. Use pure alcohol (do not use rubbing alcohol, it is too harsh and drying for face and hair treatments and it smells so strong that it will overpower any attempts of scenting). Place on a sunny window sill and swirl gently every day for 4–6 weeks; strain off herbs or flowers and decant into a sterilized tinted bottle.

Obesity and the Liver, Kidney, Heart Disease and Diabetes

As you read about the conditions and indications these herbal medicines can potentially treat, you may be wondering what all that has to do with you. You haven't heard you have trouble with your liver or kidneys for example. Maybe you haven't even thought about your kidney and liver. Let sleeping dogs lie, so to speak. High HDL and blood pressure – not me, you say.

Obesity, that word stings the tongue as it comes out. We don't like to think of ourselves as obese yet you only need to be over 20% of your ideal body weight to be obese. When a woman has more than 30% body fat or a man has over 25% body fat they are considered obese. You can also define obesity by figuring out your body mass index or BMI. The BMI is a mathematical formula based on your height and weight. Starting this weight-loss journey, my BMI was a whopping 35! Some of you reading this already know you fall into this category and some of you are hiding from the fact. It needs to be faced directly, here and now, so that you can move on in a healthier fashion.

When you are obese the following ailments arise:

- Raised blood cholesterol and triglyceride levels
- Reduced "good" HDL cholesterol. HDL cholesterol is linked with lower heart disease and stroke risk, so low LDL tends to raise the risk
- Increase in blood pressure
- Development of diabetes. In some people
- Increased risk of heart attack from diabetes

Usually the domain of alcoholics, there is also a nonalcoholic fatty liver disease known as NAFLD that is very dangerous to your health. If you have an excess of belly fat, you could be in danger of developing a form of this. A wide array of diseases fall under the spectrum of NAFLD:

- Fatty liver: accumulation of fat in the liver, also called steatosis
- Nonalcoholic steatohepatitis, also referred to as NASH, is fat in the liver that causes liver inflammation
- Cirrhosis: permanent advanced, advanced scarring of the liver resulting from chronic inflammation of the liver

NOTE: THE DIABETES CONNECTION

Many types of NFLD come from insulin resistance which is closely
related back to obesity. All the stages of NFLD are believed to be due
to insulin resistance, which is closely related to obesity. The larger you
are by weight and lie size, the greater weight-wise liver, the greater the
chances of liver damage.

Lighten Your Load: Helpful and Clarifying Plants

Let's face it, most of us are living in urban or suburban environments.
For us, gathering wild foods is a far away notion. Still, wild plants
are ornery and they do not limit themselves to the far away. Weeds
that you don't even plant yourself are also healing herbs that can
help you with this work you've undertaken.

Wild Medicines

Some nourishing and strengthening herbs built to address the
issues arising out of being overweight or obese, will pop up, of their
own volition in your yard and elsewhere. They are full of nutrients
and include:

Burdock Root

One of my favorite of all herbs, this plant grows as an ornery
weed in the garden. The root is edible and can be chopped up and
simmered, then eaten like oatmeal. It is a blood purifying weed
that contains vitamin A and C. It has been used in Native American
medicine, by the Chinese historically and then by European settlers
for vitality, health, digestion and the gas we get from suddenly
eating lots of fruits and raw vegetable, while slimming. It reduces

blood sugar, strengthens urinary and kidney function (important when consuming a lot of water). Burdock root reduces swelling and painful joints because it is an anti-inflammatory.

Put 1 teaspoon of the dried root in 8 ounces of water and simmer 10–15 minutes. Strain, sweetened with maple syrup or honey if desired.

Dandelion

This is so omnipresent, particularly in urban areas, they need no introduction. While we are busy getting rid of dandelions, they are prepared to help you heal if you let them. If you are struggling with your weight, and I assume you are, or you wouldn't be reading this book this far in, this is a good weed to add to your arsenal. It regulates blood sugar for those with diabetes, lowers cholesterol, and is an anti-inflammatory that relieves pain and swelling because of the high amounts of essential fatty acids they contain.

Drink as a tea of the roots (see burdock root) or eat simmered like kale.

Chickweed

Chickweed is an age-old obesity-fighting herb beloved by herbalists to treat those suffering with being overweight. It is a blood cleansing herb with mild laxative actions. It is a blood cleansing herb with mild laxative actions. It is also an anti-inflammatory.

Red Clover

You can't stop red clover from growing. It grows wherever it wants. That can work out in your favor because this is a nutritious and supportive weed. Red Clover has the richest source of isoflavones (a water-soluble estrogen-like chemical). It is known to lower cholesterol and supports healthy urine production. Red Clover contains chromium which is used to support weight-loss and contains magnesium, a natural pain-reliever and sleep aid. It also contains niacin, phosphorus, potassium, thiamine and Vitamin C.

Lambs-quarter

This delightful and delicate weed grows in most yards. It is cleansing and purifying. It will restore nutrients that have been depleted. You can add the leaves and flowers to salads, smoothies, juices, soups and sautés.

Milk Thistle

This is my go-to herb for spring cleansing the body and detoxification. Milk Thistle enjoys a lengthy history in folk medicine and it has caught the eye of the medication establishment. It is being investigated for helping with cholesterol and even cancer. Milk Thistle is best known for helping cleanse and tone the liver. It is used in the treatment of cirrhosis of the liver as well as for toxin-induced liver damage and even mushroom poisoning.

Milk Thistle is taken as a tincture because it is difficult to extract or decoct into a tea. The seeds are the most beneficial part. They can also be ground (1 teaspoon) and added to any type of smoothie. Some people take them in capsule form, taking 100–250 mg per day.

Purslane

In Malawi, Purslane is called: Buttocks of the Wife of the Chief.

It has more Omega-3 fatty acids as any other green plant. It tastes a little like arugula, with a bitter bite. It is widely eaten in Crete and Uzbekistan. This weed, also called hogweed can be eaten in salad. It is rich in beta-carotene.

NOTE

You should check with your naturopath or holistic health doctor for interactions or counter indication with any of these herbs. Wild Medicine is still medicine.

MORTAR and PESTLE

A grinding tool used since ancient times by herbalists, witches, healers, midwives and cooks. It consists of a bowl (the mortar) and a crushing wand to use against the interior of the bowl (the pestle). Mortar and pestle can be used to grind rough spices, herbs, roots and berries. It is popularly used today to create guacamole and all types of flours. This is an essential healers' tool.

Grandmother of the Forest: Baba Yaga

Baba Yaga is a goddess from Russian that you will find in the forest. Baba Yaga is Grandmother of the Forest. Among other creatures, she is associated with crows, ravens, owls and dragons. Careful! Baba Yaga is rightfully feared – she is fierce. She flies around on a mortar, steered by a pestle. Secretive as she is, she sweeps away all traces of her path with a broom.

She has iron teeth, some of which protrude like tusks. She has fingers that flare out with ends of bear claws and she is partial to skulls and bones. Baba Yaga wears a necklace of skulls. Her yard is fenced with a collection of different sorts of animal bones. The dominant feature of her hut is the hearth, where a magical cauldron of renewal sits ready to usher in change.

The fierce goddess, Baba Yaga, has no patience, for whining or making excuses, a pre-occupation for many a would-be slimmer. Go to Baba Yaga when you are looking for just the right herbal cure for the symptom, helping to weigh you down.

So many books that seek to help you lose weight are focused around food. You begin to think you eat too much and that is what gets you in trouble. Yes and no. It's as much what you eat as it is what is eating away at you, slowly but surely and that mental connection gets little attention.

Well how about you try a new tactic? Baba Yaga loves to eat. If you trust yourself enough, create a lavish gourmet feast to honor Baba Yaga. Unload the things you can no longer eat on her altar. Petition her help, with helping you discover just the right botanical cure for what's eating at you.

You can also try this chant to find inner peace, when you fear consumption will get the best of you:

Peace Chant

May the heaven be peaceful
May the earth be free from disturbance
May the vast atmosphere be calm
May the flowing waters be soothing
and all the plants and herbs prove beneficial to us.

From: Atharva Veda. XIX. 9. 1

Not one for chanting? Perhaps you'd like to say this prayer. Sit down, quiet your mind say this prayer from your heart:

Metta or Loving-Kindness Prayer Practice (Buddhist)

May I be free from fear
May I be free from suffering
May I be happy
May I be filled with loving-kindness

Baba Yaga's Altar

You might be wondering why I am putting you in touch with such fierce goddesses. It is because transformation can be an ugly and distressing process. Implicit within it is destruction, death and rebirth – all this to change the way you are currently existing. We are not messing around are we? This is powerful work and for that we need powerful spiritual assistance.

Directions

1. Lay out a gorgeous bright orange cloth (like the sun), to represent Baba Yaga's planet.
2. Put an elaborate European dragon on the cloth next to Poppies, black sunflowers or wild flowers.
3. Leave her some rye bread, Russian black tea, tobacco (for the pipe she smokes) and a shot of vodka.
4. Lay corn sheaths near the food, drink and tobacco.

NOTE

Petition Baba Yaga when you mean it and want her powerful guidance. Maintain your altar to her by cleaning it and replenishing it often, so as not to anger her.

Baba Yaga's Cottage of Natural Remedies

In thinking of the wisdom of Baba Yaga that you have obtained from engaging and invoking her spirit at the altar, consider her cottage in the birch forest and how it holds remedies important to your weight-loss journey. Go into the cottage respectfully. Look in her imaginary cupboards. This is what you're likely to find for our work here:

Appetite Suppressants

Chia Seeds

Flaxseed

Water Retention Aids

Uva Ursi

Cranberries

Parsley

Regularity and Constipation Aids

Flax tea

Prune Juice

Senna

Banana

Satiety Aids

Coconut oil

Avocados

Nuts

Energizing Fat Busters

Lemon

Water

Green Tea

Cayenne

Cinnamon

Digestive Aids

Ginger

Papaya

Pineapple

Fennel Seeds

Bad Mood Tamers

Oat Straw

Linden Flowers

Pasque Flowers

Cerridwin and her Cauldron of Knowledge

Cerridwin is a very important Celtic Mother Goddess from Wales. She is significant to your conversation here because she is an adept herbalist who brews an infinite cauldron of knowledge. Just as important for us in our weight-loss journey is her fluidity and ability to change her appearance. At will Cerridwin can change herself, shape shifting into different forms – one of her favorites is that of a white sow or female pig.

Pigs represent good fortune and spiritual enrichment. Cerridwin possesses creativity and deep knowledge. She is a source of inspiration and brings luck and good fortune with her, wherever she goes. I would like you to pay homage to Cerridwin's many attributes, and for you to have the ability to invoke her knowledge, whenever needed. For that, we need to do a special project.

I know that some of you will not consider yourselves creative. Others feel too mired in the diet plan to expend any extra energy. Trust me, though this project will work many wonders, much like Cerridwin herself.

MATERIALS NEEDED

Flour

Water

Sugar

Pot

Bowl

Newspaper

Acrylic Polymer Medium or Modge Podge

White Paint

Tacky Craft Glue

(Optional: decorative materials such as feathers, beads, markers)

Papier Mache Recipe

1 cups all-purpose flour

4 cups cold water

4 cups boiling water

½ cup sugar

Combine the flour and cold water in a large bowl. Add this mixture to a saucepan of boiling water. Bring to a boil. Remove from heat and stir in the sugar. Cool; (it will thicken as it cools).

NOTE

Can be stored in the refrigerator for a few days if needed in a covered container.

Directions

1. Cover a 12″ balloon with a layers of papier mache. Tie the balloon tightly, so the balloon stays inflated while drying.

2. Cover the balloon with a second layer of newspaper strips, preferably in the opposite direction.

3. Smooth out the body and to whiten the overall color and strengthen Cerridwin, cover the balloon with a layer of the papier mache using white paper towel strips.

4. For Cerridwin's feet, take small Dixie Cups (the 2″ tall bathroom) and glue them to the bottom of the balloon.

5. Add another Dixie Cup over the knot of the balloon for the snout. Cut and glue the curved part of a cup and use it for the ears.

6. Make one more paper towel covering, making sure they cover the ears, nose and feet of their pig.

7. Paint Cerridwin white, but add any decorations you wish. After the paint dries, cut the coin slots with a razor knife and apply acrylic polymer medium (glossy) to Cerridwin to make her durable, strong and shiny.

8. Use your Cerridwin piggy bank icon to reward yourself. Put money inside the slot in the form of coins. If you prefer not to fill her with money, write good thoughts about your journey on a piece of paper whenever you meet your different weight-loss milestones and goals, fold it small and flat and stuff it into Cerridwin. When you are finished, you should either have a good stash of money saved up with which you can do something special or a wonderful collection of good thoughts to put into your journal. These thoughts are documentation of the various steps you took to meet your goals.

CHAPTER 3

Fruitful Harvest: Elixirs from the Garden of Eden

I am a magical herbalist and aromatherapist. What that means is, I believe in and utilize the magical and spiritual qualities of herbs, using them to treat the conditions of the mind, body and spirit. As an aromatherapist, I utilize scent, be it from essential oil, absolutes or hydrosol for the purposes of healing.

Back in 1999, I started my own small natural product company called Almost Edible Natural Products. Using my knowledge of magical herbalism and aromatherapy, I make sachets, incense, potpourri, bath soaks, body butters and soaps.

In this chapter, I share ways you can employ magical herbalism and aromatherapy in your weight-loss journey. You will find in these next pages a focus on essential oils, the medicinal extracts derived from plants. This is the space where I share how essential oils can be employed in ways as diverse as increasing circulation to reducing cellulite.

We enter this chapter through the Garden of Eden. This is the place I want you to visualize filled with earthly delights. Gardens are the epicenter of healing. You can reduce your body through what you grow and harvest. Growing healing herbs not only provides much needed exercise but it also soothes the anxiety that builds up in you, causing unhealthy behaviors like overeating to manifest. We will consult the gods, goddesses and spirits of the plants along the way. We will be practicing internalizing their messages through affirmations, incantation, invocation and the creation of altars.

Speaking of creativity, you will also make useful elixirs, potions and brews, to aid your weight-loss, starting now, with Czech goddess Jezibaba.

Jezibaba the Granny Witch

Jezibaba, the Granny Witch of the forest is likely related to Baba Yaga, whose wisdom proved inspirational in the previous chapter. The two live in similar spaces – they both love the woods. Jezibaba lives near a lake and water is her element.

We are stopping by her cottage first because Jezibaba is a master herbalist and we are going to be working with her medicines. It is very helpful if you petition her at the beginning of your magical herbalism work. This goddess, though not as fierce as Baba Yaga, doesn't like to be played with.

We are about the head (the mind in our triangle of mind, body and spirit) most of the time. Why not head south and work on our feet? Part of compulsive eating stems from being stressed out. How about you make yourself a foot soak and then carry on reading?

Jezibaba's Foot Potion

Ah, the pleasures of simple relaxation. When I read about weight-loss, sometimes when I'm not ready for the prospect or work required, I get stressed out and in the past, I would mindlessly munch on cookies or brownies while doing the reading. I had it bad, I admit.

You might not have thought about it before but self-care and loving acts of self-kindness, can aid your weight-loss. Use the time while soaking your feet to refresh, recharge and relax. Try some sort of foot soak at least once a week. This makes a welcomed treat when you are celebrating meeting one of your milestones.

Ingredients and Equipment

½ cup lavender buds
5 drops lavender essential oil
Handful dried peppermint leaves
3 drops peppermint essential oil
Very Warm Water (use spring water if possible)
Basin or bath tub

1. Light a blue candle to lend an atmosphere of peace and tranquility.
2. Ask Jezibaba to bless all your ingredients and your basin or tub with the ability to be relaxing and recharging. Look at each element of this recipe as you ask for her assistance.
3. Put the water in the basin or run a shallow foot bath in the tub.
4. Warm your hands with the energy from the candle.

5. Take the lavender buds in your warmed hands and rub the buds between your palms. This action releases the medicinal essential oils.

6. Repeat this process with the peppermint leaves.

7. (As you rub the herbs with your warmed hands, imagine Jezibaba looking out over her lake from the windows of her cottage. Imagine how relaxed and connected to the universe she feels as she reflects on her element).

8. Cup your hands and take a deep inhalation of the buds and leaves.

9. With your exhale, release the herbs into the water.

10. Now, concentrate your energies on the essential oil bottles.

11. Drop the oils into the herbal water, while imagining this is the water of Jezibaba's realm.

12. Take slow, meditative breaths with each drop.

13. Wash your feet first and them pat them dry (not in the basin but elsewhere).

14. Now put your feet into the Jezibaba Foot Potion and relax for 10–20 minutes.

HYGIA, GODDESS of HYGIENE

Hygeia is the Greek Goddess of health and health. We have derived the name hygiene from her name. She was venerated in temples and continues to be important to our wellbeing.

Paying Attention to Hygiene

I am only going to talk about water in these chapters in two ways because later, we will be working the element of water. Early on though, we need to discuss hygiene. Hygiene in lieu of Goddess Hygeia, and hydrosols useful to your weight-loss are the ways we will discuss water right now.

We don't always like to go there, talking about hygiene but it is important, as you are losing weight. You should be drinking at least eight glasses of water of 8 ounces per glass. You will also most likely be drinking the herbal teas suggested in this book. That, in and of itself, is a huge portion of water consumed every day, which is not to mention the water you are getting from fresh fruits and your homemade soups. This water consumption means you will be going to the bathroom, and I do mean, a lot, all day and for some of you even during the night.

Stay careful and attentive to your body's cleanliness. I'm serious. Hygeia warns you to wipe yourself from front to back, always – don't get sloppy just because you are running back and forth to the bathroom frequently. If you don't you will surely get a painful urinary tract infection from the bacteria you've spread. She goes on to say, "Wash your hands often and thoroughly, just with a good herbal soap, since you will frequently be preparing herbal solutions and cutting up whole foods."

Loving Yourself with Anaisu Pye's Assistance

Called a lwa and metresa (female lwa/mistress), Anaisa Pye is Queen of Love in the 21 Divisions. She is highly thought of in the

Dominican Republic and in Gaga, a Vodou-inspired path brought there by Haitians.

A jealous and possessive lwa/metresa, Anaisa Pye is not to be trifled with in the same way you don't play around with Jezibaba or Baba Yaga. If you decide to invoke her or build an altar for her, be dedicated and serious. She doesn't like to share space with other female lwa either, so make hers a dedicated space.

I want to get you to invite Anaisa Pye into your spiritual weight-loss practice, at this particular point because she cultivates beauty, desirability and reigns over domestic issues. She is also very fond of scent and we are going to be getting into essential oils. She can help you improve your way of imagining yourself. Attraction that comes from within acceptance of yourself is the sexiest most attractive type of all. This spirit loves fine scents and perfumery thus she is the gate through which we will approach aromatherapy.

---

21 DIVISIONS

The 21 Divisions or Las 21 Divisiones also called Dominican Vodou and Los Misterios is a spiritual path from the Dominican Republic. This religious practice is eclectic, blending elements of Yoruba practices of Nigerian, Taino Indian beliefs (indigenous people), Kongo, Benin, Haitian Vodou and Catholicism.

Anaisa Pye Altar

Remember to only build this altar, if you are going to dutifully maintain it and you are not going to pay homage to any other metresa. Anaisu Pye and her effects on your life can be a long lasting presence.

WHAT YOU NEED

A shiny pink cloth that shimmers in the light

St. Anne and Archangel Michael candle

Champagne or Belgian Beer in a champagne glass

A pink rose in a vase with water

5 beeswax votive candles

Your favorite perfume or perfumed oil

Directions

1. Spread the cloth on a mantel.
2. Place the St. Anne and Archangel Michael candle in the center.
3. Make a circle around the tall candles out of the votive candles.
4. Put the champagne glass inside the circle.
5. Pour the champagne or beer into the glass.
6. Drop your perfume into the glass and swirl gently to mix.
7. Put some perfume on yourself.
8. Light all candles when you are seeking to love yourself and to express that loving acceptance to others.

Aromatherapy and Essential Oils

Aromatherapy is the art and science of healing with aromatic plants. The primary vehicle for providing aromatherapy is using essential oils. I told you about my aromatherapeutic blends at the beginning of this chapter. Essential oils are the essence of the plant extracted to yield concentrated oil. Within that essence there are volatile oils, phyto-nutrients and other valuable medicinal substances called chemical constituents. Aroma releases certain chemical reactions in the brain. Aromas can control or stimulate appetite, depending on the plant, and they also control certain emotions.

Fragrance can address and create specific states of mind. You will see shortly how, aromatherapy can be received through scented candles like lavender or rose candles for example; bath salts, lotions and creams, sachets, bath soaks, sprays, ointments, teas, fire, heat elements and from being diluted in a carrier oil and applied to the skin, especially the pulse points or through massage. We turn now to the aromatherapeutic benefits of essential oils when it comes to supporting weight-loss.

Herbal Essential Oils for Weight-loss Support

Basil (*Ocimum basilicum*) reduces stressful feelings, stimulant, tonic, calming, eases nervousness and acts as an antidepressant.

Bergamot (*Citrus aurantium var. bergamia*) fights depression, combats fear, eases nervous tension and stress and addresses eating disorders.

Clary sage (*Salvia sclarea*) is a sedative that fights nervousness, acts as antidepressant and euphoric; it also alleviates tension and stress.

Cypress (*Cupressus sempervirens*) eases the way through difficult lifestyle changes, calms anger and irritability, de-stresses, and relieves pain and suffering. Avoid during pregnancy

Dill (*Anethum sowa*) (*A. graveolens*) is a calming, sedative that helps when you are feeling overwhelmed; dill oil alleviates gas and constipation.

Sweet Fennel (*Foeniculum vulgare var. dulce*) lends longevity, courage and strength; laxative, diuretic, stimulant and tonic which reduces obesity. *Avoid with certain cancers, pregnancy, breast feeding and epilepsy.

Grapefruit (*Citrus paradise; Citrus racemosa*) cleansing; treats sluggish lymph drainage, fat metabolizing, fights obesity and is brightening to the spirits. *Can irritate skin if exposed for long periods of time to the sun.

Jasmine (*Jasminum Gradiflora syn. officinalis*) deeply relaxing, antidepressant, sedative, soothing; jasmine instills confidence. Not to be used during pregnancy.

Juniper (*Juniperus communis*) helps alleviate mental exhaustion, deters anxiety, helps you deal with nervous tension, fights cellulite, acts as a diuretic, is useful in the fight against obesity and it curtails the desire to over-eat.

Lavender (*Lavendula officinalis*) is used for nervous disorders, tension, hysteria, and exhaustion, stress, as an antidepressant, diuretic, sedative and a pain killer.

Lemon (*Citrus limonum*) helps the circulatory systems, boosts immunity, calming and serves as a tonic. * Not to be used before exposure to the sun.

Marjoram (*Oreganum marjorana*) is calming, addresses emotional issues, relaxing, fights anxiety; marjoram is calming and warming. *Not to be used during pregnancy.

Neroli (*Citrus aurantium var. amara; Citrus vulgaris; C. Bigardia*) fights fear and combats shock. It is deeply relaxing, quells anxiety, acts as a sedative, tonic, useful for weight-loss, eases inhibitions and insecurity, and serves as an antidepressant. Neroli relieves gas some experience when beginning a new eating plan.

Patchouli (*Pogostemon cablin; Pogostemon patchouli*) revitalizes, bring more energy, acts as an antidepressant, reduces appetite, functions as a diuretic and relieves anxiety.

Rosemary (*Rosmarinus officinalis*) is uplifting, clears the mind, sharpens awareness, reduces fatigue, addresses nervous disorders and de-stresses. * Should not be used in pregnancy or when high blood pressure is an issue.

Spearmint (*Methna Spicata*) is stimulating, uplifts spirits, relieves gas and constipation, fights fatigue, and addresses nervousness and stress.

Thyme (*Thymus bulgaris*) relieves nervousness, increases concentration and energy, acts as an antidepressant. Thyme is a stimulant that decreases exhaustion. *Not to be used in pregnancy, with epilepsy or with high blood pressure; should be used in low concentrations.

Ylang, Ylang (*Cananga odorata)* reduces nervousness and treats fragile nerves, acts as a sedative, antidepressant and euphoric.

Its Elemental: Receiving Aromatherapy

Essential oils should always be taken with a heart filled with gratitude for the fruitful harvest presented by Mama Earth. Gratitude can be expressed with a few simple but direct words expressed out loud in the form of prayer. In addition, the elements play an important role in the delivery of essential oils as aromatherapy. Fire (heat), water and air are the chief ways of administering essential oils to achieve the desired benefits.

Water

Sitz bath: fill tub to navel or hips; add 2–3 drops of your preferred essential oil to the water; swirl with your hand or a metal spoon to disperse.

Foot soak: soak feet for 20 minutes in a basin of hot water to which you've added 2–6 drops of essential oils.

Hand soak: soak hands for 20 minutes in a shallow pan of hot water to which you've added 3–4 drops of essential oils.

Shower: after washing and rinsing yourself place 8 drops of your favorite essential oils (can be a blend) onto wash cloth; breathe in the aromatic steam.

Bowl: 2–9 drops placed in a large bowl of boiling water; the aroma is inhaled for 5 minutes.

Fire

Fireplace: place 1 drop of woodsy essential oil such as cypress or juniper on a log. Let soak for a half hour before lighting.

Light bulb: using a light bulb diffuser follow manufacturer's directions.

CARRIER OILS

Essential oils are strong concentrations of a plant's volatile oils and chemical constituents. Therefore, they should be diluted before using directly on skin. Here are some oils to consider using as carrier or base oils to dilute your essential oils:

*All oils must be cold pressed for added purity and organic is preferred.

- Sweet almond oil
- Apricot kernel oil
- Grape seed oil
- Sunflower oil
- Corn oil
- Safflower oil

Radiator: soak a cotton ball with 2–8 drops of essential oil blend of your choice.

Candle: light candle; let burn for a few minutes; drop 1–2 drops of essential oil into the melted wax.

Lotus Oil

There is plenty of mystique around the lotus flower throughout the world, particularly in Asia where it features prominently in the meditative mandalas. The scent and physical structure of the flower is likened to hyacinth, and to the sexuality of women. The white lotus, *Nymphaea lotus L.*, only blooms at night. Lotus has been synonymous with love and became the focus for the mythic tales of creation--after all it grows in water, the domain of the emotions. The plant's oils are slightly narcotic, causing deep sedation and relaxation.

Other

Tissue or handkerchief: add 1 drop of essential oil to hanky or tissue and inhale for 5 minutes.

Massage: Add 5 drops of essential oil per teaspoon of carrier oil.

Cleansing the Crown: Working Mae Thoranee

The mind, body, spirit paradigm must always be at the forefront of your mind, as you attempt the ambitious goal of losing weight and keeping it off. The mind and spirit play an important role in changing the shape and form of your body. This is a different way of thinking; I know because usually books about slimming down focus on the body and on food. The main mental function discussed is will power.

In many healing traditions around the world, the act of washing the head, or what I like to refer to as the crown, brings about a sense of wellbeing and restores healthy balance. Keeping that in mind, we move on to the goddess Mae Thoranee.

Mae Thoranee, is the Earth Mother of Thailand. She guards the earth, protecting its cattle and people. Mae Thoranee is the most popular Thai deity.

This goddess stands for all the positive qualities of the earth. She is kind, generous, and divinely feminine. She protects against spiritual danger we encounter through struggles with sugar and carbohydrate addiction, as well as offering strength to make it through temptations.

Mae Thoranee's power and willingness to lend her mothering power to this journey you have undertaken cannot be underestimated. For one thing, she can banish devilish demons and malevolent spirits. Her energy is particularly well suited to addictions, compulsions and food obsessions.

She enjoys water, rice, sugar, betel nuts, flowers, incense and candles, so we will use some of her choice offerings in your invocation ritual.

Creative Visualization

First though, you must fix her in your mind's eye. She is primordial like all Earth Mothers. Her original manifestation was as a black-skinned, green-hair woman. The black skin represents the fertility of healthy soil and the green hair is what grows from the soil. Her eyes are like two, stunningly beautiful blue lotuses, representing a crystal-clear sky. Often nowadays, she is pictured as a black-haired, blue-eyed Thai woman, whose hair is so long, it trails the ground.

Mae Thoranee is known to squeeze and twist her luxuriously long hair to release the water from it. Considering her iconography, attributes, appearance and fighting spirit, I have designed the following cleansing ritual for you to do, as you invoke her spirit.

As you conduct this personal ritual focus on releasing your inner demons, which include ills Mae Thoranee loves to address:

- Compulsions
- Addictions
- Obsessions

This is no Earth Mama for the faint of heart; indeed, if one exists, I do not know her. Mae Thoranee has traditionally been invoked by soldiers going into battle. She oversees planting of rice, a symbol of fertility, and at harvest. This is a serious, well-equipped, reinforcing goddess, which must be respected, honored and invoked, as you do your own kind of serious battle in the hopes of effecting a lasting change.

Moving Mae Thoranee Meditation

1. When you are lying in bed, I want you to visualize Mae Thoranee. Ask her to give you inner strength and the will to meet your goals for the day.
2. As you come to the side of the bed, made sure your feet are bare.
3. Call out to Mae Thoranee to get her attention before your feet touch the ground.
4. When your feet touch the ground, imagine you are standing on the shoulders of the original black-skinned, green-haired, blue-eyed Mae Thoranee.
5. Thank her from deep in your heart for standing next to you, supporting you on this day in your journey.

Invoking the Thai Earth Goddess: Cleansing the Crown

1 cup rice milk
6 drops blue lotus oil

1. Bring your image of the long-haired Mae Thoranee with you to the shower.

2. Wash your hair with your favorite shampoo.
3. As you squeeze out your hair, imagine you are banishing distractions, preventing you from meeting your goals.
4. As the water escapes from your hair and drains, imagine it is taking away any hesitance or fear in your head.
5. Repeat this process, continuing your focus on banishing your distractions and excuses as well.
6. Watch as the water goes down your body and into the drain. Understand that rice is an offering to Mae Thoranee.

Now, take your cup of rice milk mixed with blue lotus oil, and whisper Mae Thoranee's name three times into the cup.

1. Pour this blessed milk over the top of your hair.
2. Imagine Mae Thoranee imbuing you with strength; showering you with protection.
3. Rinse your hair thoroughly.
4. Squeeze it out carefully as you continue your thoughts of banishing the demons that haunt you.
5. Pat yourself dry and fasten a towel around your head.
6. You are sealing in Earth Mother Mae Thoranee's protective energy.

To complete this work, pat blue lotus oil on your pulse points, thinking of re-visioning yourself the way you want to be.

Mae Thoranee Libation

The ritual I gave previously works well if you have long dread locks like I did, or very long hair, at the least below the shoulders. If you have short hair or are bald it isn't going to work for you. Instead, try this libation.

LIBATIONS

A libation is the purposeful pouring of sacred liquid such as floral water, holy, rain or plain water on the Earth Mama, to invoke spirits or ancestors of the earth.

Ingredients

Tall glass of spring water
Mound of beautiful, fertile soil

1. Cup the container of water in your hands.
2. Whisper your addiction, compulsion and/or obsession that has led to your weight gain into the glass.
3. Exhale into the glass of water completely expelling your worries with your complete expulsion of air.
4. Pour the water onto the mound of earth while imagining you are turning your worries and anxiety over to Earth Mother Mae Thoranee.

Easy Slimming Recipes to Soothe the Mind, Body and Spirit

Toning Oils for the Bath

3 drops each grapefruit, basil and lavender essential oils.

Metabolize Your Fat Massage

10 drops each: fennel, lavender, juniper or basil, cypress, grapefruit, added to 6 teaspoons carrier oil from list provided.

Water Weight Reduction Shower

2 drops cypress, 2 drops lemon, 4 drops grapefruit added to wash cloth and inhaled 5 minutes with shower running.

Lift Your Spirits Candle

Add 1 drop neroli and 1 drop lavender to melted candle wax, burn candle and enjoy!

A Whiff of Self Confidence

Add 1 drop of neroli to your handkerchief or tissue. Inhale for about 5 minutes.

Earth Mama has so many prized solutions to weight-loss, take the elixirs in the form of essential oils, presented here for an example. Essential oils can be used in many ways to creatively and spiritually support your weight-loss efforts. Engaging the earth, its beings, deities and spirits through acts of invocation, petition and offering further enhance the magical potential of essential oils. In the next chapter, we continue to explore elixirs from nature and the spirits that bless them; this time focusing in on the healing medicines from flowers.

CHAPTER 4

Flowers: Gentle and Fragrant Healers

Walking the Path of Enchantment and Beauty

Throughout history flowers and other plant parts such as roots, berries, bark, leaves, buds and even moss, have served many vital functions that support wellness. Today they continue to have an important role in our lives. Flowers for example, are given to offer well wishes, for celebrations, to help someone get well, as a thank you and an expression of love. These methods of giving have a spiritual component that when coupled with the plethora of Earth Mama's offerings yield a potent cure. We know fruits, leaves, roots, berries, barks, moss are healers, this chapter shows how you can employ flowers, the gods, goddesses and spirits of flowers to work together to support the fight against obesity and facilitate weight-loss.

Floral Cures

A beautiful arrangement of flowers can do more than uplift the spirits; it can take your breath away, filling the room with its exotic perfume. Perfumes with floral notes, take the mind on a romantic journey into the land of various gods and goddesses which we will explore in a few pages. At the same time, flower medicine doesn't have to be fragrant to have healing effects or help with your weighty issues. Take flower essences for an example. Flower essences attack many of the underlying causes that lead us to becoming overweight. True, one issue with obesity is the calculation of calories in, calories out, but there is also the rationale behind the reasons why we consume too many calories. Some of the reasons flowers can address are: boredom, resentment, anger, hostility, fear, anxiety, loss of control, shock, apathy, addiction, and feeling overwhelmed or hopeless.

Goddess Flora: Essence of Flowers

Before honing in on flower essences, let's stop in to see the Essence of Flowers in goddess form, Goddess Flora. Flora is the deity of blooming flowers. This goddess was celebrated in Rome during the celebration in her name, called Floralia.

- Flora speaks to us about our potential, to blossom and flower, becoming all that we hope to be.
- As you set your goals and work towards them, always keep this flower goddess close to the heart.
- Flora's wisdom asks us to honor where we are today – to be of the moment.

- She also asks us to embrace our bodies, love our curves and celebrate ourselves as we are.
- Flora is the name given to plants of the natural world.
- She is intimately tied to Earth Mama and her gifts.

Engaging with Flora

1. Today, why not bring in a bunch of flowers – gather them from the garden, forest, meadow (if you are so fortunate) or from the florist.
2. Gaze upon your flowers, noticing how beautiful they are and how they fill your senses, most likely even better than food.
3. Put a few blossoms in your pocket or bra.
4. Carry Flora and her promise of your meeting your goals, around with you today.

Flower Essences

Flower essences are, as they sound, the essence of specific flowers. They are the essences of Flora and other gods and goddesses you are about to work with. The essence of flowers is obtained primarily from steeping them under the heat of the sun or using a boiling method. Any of you involved with magical spiritual paths will immediately recognize the spiritual significance of using the elements of fire and water, coupled with the power of Father Sun, to extract healing medicines, such as what is done in the process of creating flower essences.

Flower essences are odorless blends that work on a vibrational, emotional and energetic level. They are restorative treatments that help strike a balance between the mind, body and the spirit, paving the way to wellness.

Enter Dr. Bach

There are several types of flower essences. One of the most respected types was developed by Dr. Edward Bach in 1928. Dr. Bach developed a system that includes 37 types of flowers and 1 essence derived simply from rock water. Each of the flowers has medicinal properties that bring balance to various emotional states. Best of all, flower essences are gentle, non-habit forming and have no known side effects.

Bach Flower Essences support weight-loss by making subtle adjustments in the negative emotions that can lead to overeating by making subtle shifts that lead to positive thoughts. As you can see from the charts that follow, flower essences treat unique emotional states and they can be taken individually or formed into personalized combinations of up to 6 essences. The combinations are often based on self-diagnosis. To take them, 4 drops of the potion are taken under the tongue six times per day.

Bach Flower Essences are divided into categories as follows:

1. The Twelve Healers
2. The Seven Helpers
3. The Second Nineteen

The Twelve Healers

These plants are associated with specific personality types; the essences are used to counteract personality failings and promote beneficial changes. This chart lists the plant type, method of extraction, personality type, virtue and downfall or failing of each personality type.

The Twelve Healers Chart

Plant	Method	Personality	Virtue	Failing
Agrimony	sun	torment	stillness	torture
Centaury	sun	servant	strength	weak
Cerato	sun	foolish	wisdom	self-distrusting
Chicory	sun	demanding	love	self-pitying
Clematis	sun	dreamer	gentleness	indifference
Gentian	sun	depressed	understanding	disconnected
Impatiens	sun	irritable	forgiveness	impatient
Mimulus	sun	nervous fear	sympathy	fearful
Rock Rose	sun	terrified	courage	terrified
Scieranthus	sun	indecision	steadfastness	full of indecision
Vervain	sun	fervent	tolerance	intense
Water Violet	sun	isolated	joy	aloof

The Seven Helpers

Recommended by Dr. Bach for patients with habitual conditions, the Seven Helpers are for a patient whose true nature is hidden and does not fit easily into the categories set by the twelve healers.

Seven Helpers Chart

Plant	Method	Chronic Condition
Gorse	sun	hopelessness
Heather	sun	talkative
Oak	sun	persevering
Olive	sun	exhaustion
Vine	sun	domineering
Wild oat	sun	lack of direction
Rock water	none	strict idealist

The Second Nineteen Chart

Plant	Method	Emotional State
Aspen	boiling	unreasonable fears
Beech	boiling	critical
Chestnut bud	boiling	unable to learn from mistakes
Cherry Plum	boiling	loss of control
Crab Apple	boiling	feeling unclean
Elm	boiling	overwhelmed

Plant	Method	Emotional State
Holly	boiling	anger and hatred
Honeysuckle	boiling	living in the past
Hornbeam	boiling	mental or physical tiredness
Larch	boiling	loss of confidence
Mustard	boiling	depression
Pine	boiling	self-blame
Red Chestnut	boiling	imagining the worse
Star of Bethlehem	boiling	needing comfort from shock
Sweet Chestnut	boiling	utter desolation
Walnut	boiling	unsettled during life passage
White Chestnut	boiling	mental congestion
Willow	boiling	resentment and self-pity
Wild Rose	boiling	apathy

Getting Started with Flower Essences

Carefully read over the emotional states just presented. Decide what your emotional issue is. Select up to six useful remedies to treat your state of mind. Pray or meditate on the intention of improving. Then take the potion as directed on the bottle – typically six times per day, until your condition improves. Each time you take the flower essence pray or meditate for a few moments on your intention. It may take a while, just as developing the state of mind, took a while to mature into its currently troubling state. Use the power of Father Sun and Goddess Flora to propel the healing process. When you combine spirituality such as prayer or meditation with nature's gifts found in flower essences you are taking very strong medicine indeed.

Hydrosols and Floral Waters

Other healing elixirs are created from flowers. They are called variously floral waters and hydrosols. True hydrosols are by-products of the steam distillation process that produces essential oils so they are using the elements of fire and water. During the distillation of essential oils, the steam-containing oils are chilled, turning them into water with a layer of essential oil on top. The essential oils are skimmed off the top and bottled as essential oil. Only in this type of volatile condition will water mix with volatile oil, forging a single unit. The remaining water still contains small deposits of beneficial essential oils.

Hydrosols are very concentrated. They are 20–30 times more concentrated than an herbal infusion (tea). 1 teaspoon of hydrosol can be added to water and taken that way. Hydrosols can be used alone or in combination with essential oils. Hydrosols are a complimentary treatment that extends the usefulness of essential oils.

Hydrosols on their own are an economic way of healing conditions that lead to weight gain. True hydrosols are pure and should not contain preservatives, therefore they should be refrigerated. There are about 125 hydrosols. Following are some that belong in this conversation.

Hydrosols Useful for Weight-loss

Blue Sage or Green Sage (*Artemisia douglasiana*) the same herb used to create smudge sticks used for the same purpose (banishing and cleansing). Blue sage or green sage brings about mental clarity, eases mental distress; it is relaxing and a tonic.

German Chamomile (*Matricaria recutita*) **Roman Chamomile** (*Chamaemelum nobile*) relaxing, calming, eases anxiety and nervousness, and has sedative qualities.

Greenland moss (*Ledum groenlandicum*) a very powerful detoxification hydrosol. Greenland moss is an especially good treatment for addictions (such as sugar addiction and addiction to certain foods).

Juniper berry (*Juniperus communis*) used to balance water in the body.

Lavender (*Lavendula officinalis*) calms the mind and quells depression.

Linden Flowers, buds and leaves (*Tilia europaea*) are soothing, relieve anxiety, act an anti-depressant and can bring on euphoria. They are also good sleep aids.

Melissa (*Melissa officnalis*) gets rid of stressful feeling and is calming.

Neroli (*Citrus aurantium*) eases inhabitations, instills self-confidence and eases nervousness.

Orange Blossom (*Citrus aurantium*) beloved for its calming effects.

Petitgrain (*Citrux x spp. Var. Clementine*) is highly recommended for eating disorders and addictions though it must be used with care because it can increase appetite.

Rose (*Rosa damascene*) it is soothing; easing nervousness and it is very relaxing.

Rose geranium (*Pelargonium graveolens*) calms surges of energy, balances women's hormones, and acts as an antidepressant; can serve as a tonic.

Rosemary (*Rosmarinus officinalis*) revitalizes and makes a refreshing tonic.

Yarrow Flower (*Achillea millefolium*) is useful in weight-loss; used to bring balance to the body.

Smelling the Roses

One of the favored darlings of Flora's world, is the rose. Roses excite all our senses and they are useful to you in your weight-loss journey, believe it or not. Take the elixir called Attar of Roses or Rose Otto for example.

Attar of Roses (Rose Otto) is derived from the Bulgarian Damask Rose, *Rx damescena* and is pure rose oil. The early Greek healers Pliny and Galen recognized the rose as a systemic healer, meaning that it can positively impact just about all our bodily functions. Here are the ways they ease your passage as you lose weight:

- Roses are a nervine, meaning they are soothing and comforting to frayed nerves.
- Working on the mind and spirit, they generate an internal feeling of pleasantness and tolerance.

- Roses teach us to be more patient with ourselves and our process.
- They invite us to love ourselves and encourages others to be friendly and loving toward us while we are doing battle.
- Energizing roses can also calm your stomach and treat skin flair-ups.
- These beauties act as an aphrodisiac, stimulating sexual energy when we are depleted.

Pure Attar of Roses is exquisite. It is also highly concentrated. A little goes a long way which is a blessing because it is very expensive. I usually buy it in tiny vials and treat them as a self-loving and attraction drawing potion.

Rose Water

Goddess forbid, you plateau, gain weight or fall of the no-sugar wagon for a while. Roses will help you through these difficulties by encouraging self-acceptance and love. Moreover, rose water helps keep you calm and stable.

Banish the Inner Critic with Rose Water

Fill a perfume bottle or spritzer bottle with rose water.
Place this in the refrigerator.

Spray your face whenever you feel like overeating or a negative self-image asserts itself. (You may hear the voice say "this isn't working fast enough," "look at me; I'm a mess" or even "I am a failure; I can't lose weight) or are sending any other destructive messages to yourself. You must banish the inner critic demon, most practically by using affirmations.

Rose Affirmations

Place attar of roses or rose oil, on your pulse points (temple, wrists, back of the knees, etc.,) or spritz face and hair with rose water, then say each affirmation as you look in the mirror.

- I accept myself as I am and as I will be
- I surround myself with love
- I forgive myself for the mistakes I have made
- I am ready to move forward

WARNINGS

Test skin (not a known allergen).

Avoid rose products if pregnant as they stimulate the womb.

Xochiquetzal and the Simple Pleasures of Life

I'm sure you get it by now but if not, let's recap. Weight-loss is a journey. It is a state of the mind and spirit, as much is it is about the body. We don't focus in these pages on food, instead we are being mentored by a relationship to Earth Mama, her gods, goddesses, beings and spirits. Now is a good time to check in with Xochiquetzal, pronounced (Sho-CHEE-ket-zul). Aztec Goddess, Xochiquetzal reminds us to savor the sensual pleasures in life – sex, sensuality, song, dance, art, crafts and the potential within ourselves.

She is also closely associated with the Day of the Dead and one of its prized flowers, cemazuchil in the Nahuatl language or Aztec Marigold in English. Both she, and her twin brother Xochipilli (Shok-el-Peel-eh) are associated with the holiday and with cemazuchil.

Take a look at their names, starting with Xochiquetzal. The root word Xochitl (Show-CHEE-tul) means "to flower" in English. Quetzal translates to "bird of splendid feathers". So, flowering bird of splendid feathers. Xochipilli is Flower and Prince or the Flower Prince. The pair are associated with butterflies, birds, (particularly hummingbirds), flowers, sex, fertility, artisans, craftspeople and florists, dancers, singers and artists.

Goddess Xochiquetzal embodies qualities that you can use right now. She is all about potential and she always maintains a fresh vision of the world. And, don't get mistaken about her personality because of all the flowery, bird and butterfly imagery circling around in your head. This is a fierce earth goddess that turned one of her lovers into a scorpion. She makes things as she wishes them to be, with her mind.

Creativity seeps through her pores. She is one of the most creative of all the goddesses and is the creator of crafts. Xohiquetzal was the first to menstruate, having been bitten on the vagina by a bat. She didn't let that get her down. She used it to inspire life and bring creativity and vision into being.

I would like you to call upon her in the following way:

INGREDIENTS NEEDED

Self-drying white clay

Variety of paints and feathers

Small, medium and large paint brush

Hot glue gun or Tacky (craft) Glue

4 hibiscus flowers

Water

5 drops rose oil

Pot

1. Massage and work the clay gently while visualizing the beautiful and sensual Xochiquetzal. Don't massage for too long or the clay will dry out.
2. Continuing to visualize Xochiquetzal, create a vessel (a handle-less holder of precious contents).
3. Let dry for a few days.
4. Paint with lovely flowers, humming birds and butterflies
5. Adorn the rim with feathers that are vertical and stick up into the air using the glue.
6. Set aside to dry completely.

Making Xochiquetzal Essence

In this elixir, hibiscus flowers, with their deep red color and their favor in Mexico, represent the menstrual blood of Xochiquetzal, which contributes to creativity and life.

- Add the hibiscus flowers to the water in a pot.
- Cover and simmer 10 minutes.
- Strain, reserving the blood-red hibiscus brew.
- Let cool.
- Add the rose oil; swirl to mix.

Xochiquetzal Invocation and Libation

1. Raise your internal energy by invoking the goddess of dance, flowers, life and death. Do a dance outside, befitting her. If you don't feel like a dancer, spin and twirl yourself around until you feel giddy.
2. Steady yourself; take a few complete and deep breaths of the essence.
3. Pour the Xochiquetzal Essence into the vessel you have created.

Recite:

Xochiquetzal I call to you;
Xochiquetzal I honor you;
Xochiquetzal I thank you:
Help me goddess in this work I have undertaken, I implore you.
Blessed Be!

Now pour your Xochiquetzal Essence Libation on Earth Mama and reflect on the goddesses' qualities, lessons and their ability to aid your work.

Cempazuchil Brew (Aztec Marigold) (*Tagetes erecta*)

Aztec Marigold is not a true marigold annual, rather it is a more tender-leafed flower, also called calendula. This is a beautiful plant that is part of the Mexican Day of the Dead and sacred to Xochipilli. Mexicans who celebrate this holiday, treat their departed ancestors as though they are still living, bringing them their favorite foods and drinks, tobacco, flowers in a festive atmosphere. This holiday reminds us of the sacred circle of life of which Xochipilli is an important part.

Cempazuchil flowers are soothing, they bring beauty and are beautifying. Xochipilli, twin brother of Xochiquetzal, is not only highly sexual and sensual, he also favors warriors. He rules over shape-shifting as well. These aspects, battling, shape shifting and beautifying the self, come together in the following ritual bath.

Xochipilli's Aztec Marigold Brew

Ingredients

2 hands full calendula flowers
4 cups water (spring water or pure rainwater if possible)
Equipment
Pot
Colander

1. Rub the calendula flowers in your hands while drawing up an image of Xochipilli in your mind.
2. Breathe, slowly and with great intent onto the flowers before releasing them into the pot.
3. Imagine your water is rainwater (if it is not) falling from the sky onto Earth Mama's flora.
4. Turn on the flame and let the flowers simmer for 5 minutes on low heat covered.
5. Cool and drain, reserving the liquid.
6. Go the shower/bath tub area in your bathroom with the Xochipilli's Aztec Marigold Brew.
7. Take off all your clothes.
8. Open a window and feel the energy of Xochipilli rush past your body.
9. Go in the shower/tub and with the intent of embracing your inner beauty pour the brew over your head as you breathe slowly and deeply. Continue until all the brew has been used.

FLOWER TEAS

What you made is called a brew but it is also a tisane or tea. Flower teas used have been throughout the ages for their gentle, calming and mentally stabilizing, balancing abilities. Listed below are some gentle flower teas you can use to calm your nerves as you transition.

Calendula	Hibiscus	Lavender	Pasque Flower
Chamomile	Hops	Passion Flower	

Enjoy any one of these teas brewed as follows:

Purposefully add 1 teaspoons dried tea of 2 teaspoons fresh flowers to 8 ounces of water. Steep for about 5 minutes. Strain and enjoy with or without natural sweetener such as honey or agave.

Inhale the Sacred Scent of Monoi Tiare

As we come to close our enchanting flower chapter, I would like you to purchase some Monoi Tiare oil to use in ritual. First though, let's have a look at what it is. Monoi (pronounced moh-Noy) means scented oil in the R'eo-Maohi language. Tiare (pronounced tee-ray) refers to the gardenia with the Latin botanical name *Gardenia tahitensis*. *Gardenia tahitensis* is Native to the highland shores of Melanesia and Western Polynesia. It is an aboriginal introduction to the Cook Islands, French Polynesia and possibly Hawai'i with origins in the Maori culture of New Zealand.

Tiare is considered the queen of Polynesian flowers and its delicate perfume is akin to the heady scent of tuberose or species of gardenia in blossom. The flower is pure white and shaped like a pinwheel set off by dark green shiny foliage. A member of the fragrant family *Rubiaceae*, tiare, it grows on a 4-meter (approximately 13 foot) shrub and it is nontoxic. Traditionally, it is used in leis and placed behind the ears of vahines (Tahitian women) and tane (men).

Monoi Tiare is exotic, aromatic oil created by soaking the tiare (*Gardenia tahitensis*) flower in carefully refined coconut oil. Typically, the male plants are cultivated and utilized to create the scented oil since they produce profuse flowers.

Coconut oil is the foundation of Monoi Tiare. It is excellent carrier oil useful for dry, itchy and sensitive skin. Carrier oil is the vehicle oil to which other more precious oils are typically added in much smaller amounts (for example essential oils). Coconut oil is easily absorbed and astringent, thus it doesn't clog pores.

Look for the 'Appellation d'origine'

Genuine Monoi Tiare must have the label Appellation d'origine which specifies that a minimum of 15 tiare flowers are soaked in each liter of refined coconut oil. Monoi Tiare products with "appellation d'origine," are authentic and the designation is only granted to the finest products with a guarantee of superior-grade products. Appellation d'origine contributes to fair-trade and local money making enterprises of Tahitians and other groups. It recognizes local traditions and customs involved with preparing Monoi Taire. You need to pay attention to how you acquire things for this work we are undertaking. Unless you live in Hawai'i, Tahiti or New Zealand, chances are you will need to buy this oil since you won't be able to make it yourself. If you live in an area where you can make it, I encourage you to give it a try.

Monoi Tiare in Polynesian Tradition and Lore

Monoi is a traditional natural remedy beloved by various groups of Polynesians. It is the national flower and emblem of Tahiti. Monoi is a very popular remedy in Polynesian traditional medicine. It is one of the main substances in French Polynesia's traditional pharmacopoeia. It has been used to treat a variety of ailments including earaches, migraine and headaches, mosquito bites, joint and muscular pain.

It has been important in ceremony and ritual as well. Monoi is traditionally used in religious rites and ceremonies that take place in "maraes," an open-air consecrated stone temple. Maori priests of New Zealand in traditional ceremonial attire use Monoi to anoint sacred objects and to purify the offerings placed on the stone altars to honor various deities.

The flower is important part of life, death, and transition rites of passage. Used at the inception of life, following one through life's passages (which is important to what we are doing within the pages of this book), becoming an integral component of funerary rites as well. All these traditional aspects make Monoi Tiare valuable to your weight-loss journey because you are letting your old habits die off while your new healthier self is going to be reborn.

Monoi Tiare: Use it as you lose it

- As you meet your weight-loss goals follow the example of the indigenous people who love this product. They slather the bodies of newborn babies with Monoi. You can massage yourself or have someone massage you with Monoi Tiare Oil when you want to reward yourself for your hard work and welcome the changes that have come.
- During traditional funerals, the body of the deceased is embalmed and perfumed with Monoi, to ease passage to the next life. Similarly, when you are saying good-bye to your clothing that is much too large to wear, you can sprinkle it with Monoi Tiare delicately before giving it away to charity.

Section 1: Check-in

It is always a great idea to take stock. You can copy and print this self-assessment or jot down the questions and your answers in your journal. Either way, at the end of each of the four sections of the book, there will be a brief check-in for self-reflection.

1. Did you lose any weight while working through this section?
2. How much weight did you want to lose?
3. How much did you actually lose?
4. Which of the stories about ancient or indigenous wisdom resonated the most with you and why?

_____

_____

_____

_____

_____

_____

5. There are many gods, goddesses and spirits explored in the first section of this book. Which of them made the biggest impact on your weight-loss journey?

_____

_____

_____

Of all the gods, goddesses and spirits, which of them inspired you?

_____

_____

_____

Why?

_____

_____

_____

6. Did you do any of the recipes, altars, projects, affirmations or incantations?
    Of all the work you did, whether recipes, altars, projects, invocations, affirmations, meditation or incantations, which helped you with your weight-loss journey the most and why?

_____

_____

_____

_____

_____

_____

_____

Part II

Soul Healing:

Approaches from the Asian
and African Diaspora

CHAPTER 5

Ashe: Ashe within African Medicines

African Paths to Wellness

No conversation about holistic health or mind, body, and spiritual connection to weight-loss, this is where there is a special focus on healing, which is nonwestern in its orientation. As the cradle of civilization, and the home to myriad shamanic and earth-based spiritual traditions, this is where we begin our exploration into healing, which is nonwestern in its orientation. Being such an enormous, deep and broad area of wisdom, for this conversation, I am limiting the discussion to parts of West Africa, Jamaica, Cuba, Haiti and the United States. Elsewhere in this book, other African diaspora countries and their healing ways are explored.

African healing in West Africa, South America, the Caribbean and the United States has always been an integrated blend of holism. Rather than simply diagnosing symptoms of illness and dispensing pharmaceuticals, consultations have traditionally included an assessment of environmental, social, psychological and spiritual conditions. This is done in many parts of the diaspora and was even a prominent aspect of midwifery practices in the restricted spaces of the American South's plantations during enslavement. (*we prefer not to be referred to as slaves but rather as enslaved people.)

Dreams and dream interpretation play a role, attesting to African healing's mental/spiritual connection. The arts contribute to healing, as do ritual and ceremony. There is also a communal aspect to African Healing Ways that is as attractive as it is effective.

DREAM-WORKING and ANCESTOR VISITATION

Visitation with the ancestors comes about in our dreams and visions. Desiring their contact, we work diligently at inviting their energy to bless medicinal blends so that they are infused with their spirit of good will which will provide potent healing energy, growing from their connection with a wide array of entities. This is a very important facet of African-inspired healing work and holistic health.

Legba in Vodou

As we do this work, I like to envision a workable space, fixed in a certain space and time. In this chapter, we enter that liminal space which traverses spiritual and corporal realms through the gatekeepers – the Legba spirits of Haiti.

When you are about to embark on your weight-loss journey you will probably feel confused about which way to go. Furthermore, you wonder, how will I get there? You need an opening and perhaps someone to show you the way. That's why a lot of people turn to diet books. But we know about the long-term efficacy of such books, don't we? Generally, they don't offer long term results.

On a spiritual level, the Legba spirits of Vodou are a family of lwa responsible for opening the door. There are a wide variety of them. Each nancion (nation) is a distinguished group of lwa, by their nature, or the people whose spirits they serve, has its own door opening spirit called a Legba.

Legba nan Rada, has the task of opening the gate on the Great Road. That doorway permits the other spirits to participate in our rites. Without Legba nan Rada there would be no integration between the mundane and spiritual worlds.

In Haitian Vodou, the Legbas are not crossroad spirits. Sometimes called tricksters, they are also healers and lords of death. All people have a connection with the Legba spirits. All of us have access, either for opening doors or forging roads of communication and respect with their help. While Vodou is a religion, with its own priests and wise people as well as initiates, you can still interact with their spirits. It is wise, if you want to go truly in-depth to consult a Vodou priest before you start.

If you are more of a solitary practitioner, get yourself a picture of St. Anthony the Abbot, or a candle devoted to him and burn it as you reflect on the Legbas. Make sure though, that it is not a picture of St Anthony of Padua, or the type of work you are undertaking will not be effective.

Patience attracts happiness;
it brings near that which is far.

Swahili proverb

TUCK INTO LEGBA'S FAVORITE FOOD – CAYENNE

Red Peppers like cayenne, are one of the preferred foods of gatekeepers, the Legba spirits. The pepper has other health benefits too. Peppers, including those found in the popular hot sauces, are believed to curb the appetite and burn calories at the same time. A study[1] suggests peppers may help weight-loss, combined with other weight-loss efforts. Since you are already involved with such weight-loss efforts, add cayenne or other hot red peppers to your diet – it can only help assist your hard work.

---

1   Study was supported by the National Institutes of Health and McCormick Spice Company. Richard Mattes, PhD, RD, distinguished professor of foods and nutrition at Purdue University was one of the lead researchers of this study published in "Physiology & Behavior." Article source: Cayenne Pepper May Burn Calories and Curb the Appetite by Brenda Goodman, MA. Accessed 3/30/2014: http://www.webmd.com/diet/news/20110427/cayenne-pepper-may-burn-calories-curb-appetite

Come to the Plateau with Orisha Obatala

You should know by now that I am not just sitting here and idly writing this book. As I write, I am on this journey with you. I have the goal of losing close to 100 pounds. I am getting there, slowly. Currently though I've hit a plateau though, and I've been there for quite some time.

Plateaus are those times in weight-loss, when your weight hovers around the same spot on the scale. You may go up a little bit or down some. I find this is directly correlated with my menstrual cycle. Even though I am being careful with my diet and drinking lots of water and special water-releasing teas, I still get bloated. When this happens, I all but lose my cool. Anger rises in me and disappointment. I wonder, will I ever reach my lofty goal and, am I doing something wrong?

Enter orisha from the practice of Santeria, practiced quite a bit in Cuba, Obatala. Obatala is a venerated orisha, called King of *Orun* (heaven). Obatala has many *caminos* (also called avatars). I am not expecting you to become an instant practitioner of Santeria. If you do practice, this is a gentle reminder to you to petition Obatala when you reach a difficulty on your path that makes you lose your cool. If you do not practice Santeria, you can still learn a few very good lessons from learning about Obatala that will carry you through your plateau mentally and spiritually.

Are you like me, where you lose your cool when you work really hard but still plateau and don't lose weight for weeks? This is the time, when you're under duress. Many people lose hope and give up after plateauing for a sustained amount of time. During this time, it is good to learn from orisha Obatala.

Obatala is all about being calm, cool and collected. In fact, there is a Yoruban term he optimizes, *funfun*, which means cool white medicine. What some people fondly call being 'chill' or taking 'a chill pill.'

I use the words path and journey repeatedly in this book for an important reason – it is what you are on right now. We have consulted Legba nana Rada, to open the gate to our healing and weight-loss path, which leads directly to our goals. Along your path, now that you are inside the healing gates, internalize the purifying coolness of Obatala.

You can create a good picture of him from the foods he prefers. He doesn't like spicy foods or salt. Like his personality, he prefers mild tasting, calming foods that are considered by some to be bland.

I find two of his offering foods useful to introduce at this point in our conversation: coconut and cocoa butter from the cacao tree.

First let's check in with the coconut in relation to your weight-loss work, then we'll get on to cocoa butter and finally, chocolate.

THE GOOD NEWS ABOUT COCONUT OIL and OBESITY

Coconut oil can be considered a super food because of its incredible health benefits. The combination of medium length fatty acids (MCT) it contains have a very positive effect on your health.

- Encourages fat loss
- Improves brain function
- Improves healthy blood cholesterol levels

A study[1] of 40 women with a large amount of abdominal fat, were given just one ounce of coconut oil, added to their diet per day, and it led to big changes that offer all of us hope:

1. Reduction in their BMI
2. Reduced waist measurements in just 12 weeks

---

1 Lipids. 2009 Jul;44(7):593–601. doi: 10.1007/s11745-009-3306-6. Epub 2009 May 13, Effects of dietary coconut oil on the biochemical and anthropometric profiles of women presenting abdominal obesity. Assunção ML1, Ferreira HS, dos Santos AF, Cabral CR Jr, Florêncio TM.

Top 10 Evidence-Based Health Benefits of Coconut Oil, July 8, 2013, by Kris Gunnars (accessed 3/30/2014): http://authoritynutrition.com/top-10-evidence-based-health-benefits-of-coconut-oil

---

Coconut: Flesh fit for Obatala

Obatala, wise man, elder, orisha of all orishas, prefers the pure white flesh of coconut as an offering. Many may look at the stubborn brown hull and wonder how to get inside. Here are tips for selecting, opening and creating basic milk from the coconut (*Cocos nucifera*). This coconut milk has numerous purposes and can be used in your slimming efforts.

Selection – choose a coconut with chestnut brown hull, that is smooth with no apparent wholes or mold. Shake and listen for water sound. If it still contains water it will be moist and tasty.

Opening the Nut – bore two holes in the eyes using an ice pick or sharp knife. The eyes are the dark brown spots at either end of the coconut. Pour coconut water into a bowl. You can add this to your bath, beauty recipes or use it in rituals and ceremonies that honor Obatala. Hit the hull on a hard surface sharply a few times – it should crack open. You can also hit the nut with a mallet or hammer. Once cracked open, scoop out flesh which is called coconut meat, to use in recipes that follow.

Making Coconut Milk – This is a delightful addition to your stews and curries, beloved also by vegans in smoothies, soups and other dishes.

1. Heat 1½ cups of water in a kettle on medium high heat.

2. Meanwhile, grate the coconut flesh and put it in a sieve over a large bowl.

3. Just before water comes to boil, slowly pour the water over the grated coconut in the sieve a little at a time. Press the coconut meat with the back of wooden spoon.

4. Remove sieve.

5. Pour this liquid into a Pyrex measuring cup with a pouring spout (for convenience).

6. Repeat this step 3–4 times.

7. This makes about 1¼ cups rich coconut milk.

Coconut Cream: To make coconut cream, bring one and a half cups full fat milk almost to the boil. Go through steps above (making of coconut milk). Coconut cream is a bit denser, with a full-bodied, sweeter taste, just right for vegan desserts and drinks. Coconut cream works well as massage therapy oil because of its silky texture.

Toasted Coconut: Remove coconut from hull with sharp knife. Shred the coconut. Add tablespoon coconut oil to a cast iron skillet. Add pinch of sea salt if desired. Toss until medium brown. Toasted coconut is a great low-carb snack. I like to toast almonds and sunflower seeds with shredded coconut and use this as a snack food when watching movies. You can also use toasted coconut as a topping for fruit salads, yogurt or cereal.

Coconut cream works well as massage therapy oil because of its silky texture.

COCONUT and AFRICAN AMERICAN HISTORY

During early African American history, black people had many uses for coconut.

- The shell was pulverized and consumed with wine as a systemic tonic.
- It was used to accelerate movement of the blood and was deemed a favorable herb for the elders.
- The shell was made into numerous household tools such as cups, measuring containers, liquids, spoons, and small plates.
- The coconut groves were a place where enslaved people went to commune with nature and to relax in the Caribbean.[1]

1 Grime, *Ethno-botany of the Black Americans*, 106.

Cacao: Food of the Gods

Cocoa butter is one of the favored foods of orisha Obatala. It comes from the cacao tree, which is as beautiful and intriguing as it is useful. One of the top economic botanical plants, *theombroma cacao* pods yield cocoa butter, cocoa powder and that delectable confection–chocolate. I want to discuss here balancing and nurturing ways to indulge in cacao products without foiling your slimming efforts.

Cacao Trees

I recently saw a cacao tree. The tree is a remarkable sight. It has dark brown bark, resembling the color of chocolate. Curiously, white flowers grow directly from the branches and trunk of the tree. The delicate, light colored blossoms create a sharp visual contrast against the deeply colored, rough looking almost black bark. In fact, the cacao tree is one of the more unusual trees that I have seen. The scent the tree emits is quite subtle; not the rich chocolate aroma you might expect. The part of *Theobroma Cacao* utilized in cocoa butter is also edible, derived from the processed beans.

Using Cocoa Butter

Cocoa butter is a useful natural substance for vegans (those who prefer no animal products including bee's wax). An additional aspect of cocoa butter to be celebrated, is that no solvents are involved in its manufacture; it is a (human) food-grade, edible ingredient. The edible aspect is appealing and my goodness, it's so simple to use in homemade potions, creams and healing balms as you shall see.

Cocoa beans are 15% fat so they have been traditionally used as a skin softener, emollient, belly rub and soothing substance for burns.

Remember I spoke about simplicity? Well, one of my favorite ways to use cocoa butter is just to hold a small chunk of the butter in my hand as I run hot water in the bathtub. The cocoa butter melts and then acts as a skin softener as I bath.

Cocoa butter has been traditionally used in the African diaspora as a stretchmark deterrent. That is how it was first introduced to me, when I was a teenager.

> Those who are at one, regarding food, are at one in life.
>
> Malawian Proverb

Chocolate

Yes, yes, yes! Generally, we are avoiding milk chocolate, if being health-conscious. Dark chocolate, in moderation, works for some. I also advocate for the use of unsweetened cocoa powder in a fruity smoothie as a chocolate treat. How we are going to focus for the moment on chocolate, which is also derived from the pods of the cacao tree just discussed, is for nurturing yourself during your difficulties, particularly while you are in a plateau stage.

Chocolate itself is a bit newer than cocoa butter in making its way into skin and hair care scene. Chocolate is derived from the same parts of the Cacao tree but is processed adding in some other ingredients, such as milk which is also good for the hair and skin. This derivative of the cocoa pod contains flavonoids called catechins – very effective antioxidants. Lactose acid in milk has been shown to help deter wrinkles, smooth and refine skin texture. Lactose also acts as a good humectant helping retain moisture in what could be dry, winter hair. The protein chocolate contains is boosted by the milk, making it good for 'natural' hair (without chemical relaxers or permanent colorants).

DARK CHOCOLATE

Dark Chocolate, with a very high percentage of cacao has hardly any sugar. This is the type preferred for the health benefits as an occasional treat or applied externally in a spa treatment or hair care formula. Dark chocolate has 35% more of the brown paste of ground cocoa beans than other chocolate so it is a concentrated formula.

Better Than Green Tea?

Many of you are already familiar with the health benefits of green tea. You might not be familiar with the fact that cocoa has more flavonoids, which means you are gaining a huge antioxidant boost from cacao-imbued products. In fact, chocolate may well have the highest source of flavonoids available to use as a dietary ingredient – think of what that could do for you.

What's So Good about Cacao?

Nutrients:	**Minerals:**
Protein	Potassium
Riboflavin	Calcium
Vitamin A	Iron
Thiamine	Phosphorous
	Copper
	Magnesium

Savoring cacao's numerous health benefits as a nourishing treat, as well as a boon for skin and hair – adding shine, vibrancy and improving the general health.

AN IMPORTANT NOTE ABOUT CACAO, CHOCOLATE and the GLOBAL COMMUNITY

There are a wide variety of botanical-based beauty products containing cocoa butter and chocolate available in spas, salons and health food shops. As I mentioned, cacao is a huge economic blessing to some countries, unfortunately though, the way that wealth is distributed is not always fair.

It is best to buy chocolate products involved with fair-trade programs; otherwise you may be supporting child labor or even the hideous slavery industry that has cropped up in parts of Africa around the chocolate industry.

No organic chocolate products have been indicated in such unsavory schemes so buy fair-trade or organic chocolate, cocoa butter and cacao health and beauty products, avoiding the rest.

Chocolate Lovers Delight

A recent scientific study[1] in England the effects of dark chocolate on animals, humans, and in cell cultures was undertaken in the lab. The results are very encouraging for those of us chocolate lovers out there. The scientists found that eating cocoa or dark chocolate helped with the management of obesity and regulating body weight in the following ways:

- It decreased the gene expression of impaired fat synthesis
- Reduced the absorption of fats and carbohydrates
- The fat content was satisfying in a way that increases the feeling of fullness

There is even more good news. In another study[2], scientists studied women with NOW syndrome, which stands for "normal obese weight." NOW syndrome means the women had a high percentage of body fat and were at a higher risk for heart disease. Their study found eating dark chocolate could help maintain heart health in these ways:

- Causing a significant decrease in the amount of cholesterol
- Reducing markers for inflammation.
- Reduction in abdominal fat

NOTE

As I mentioned previously, the type of dark chocolate used in the study has a very high percentage of cocoa and a small amount of sugar.

---

1 "Dark Chocolate: An Obesity Paradox or a Culprit for Weight Gain?" published in the journal *Phytotherapeutic Research* and done at Queen Margaret University in Musselburgh, England.
2 The Department of Neuroscience at the University of Tor Vergata, in Rome, Italy and published in the journal *European Review for Medical and Pharmacological Sciences*.

Ayido Wedo

Phew! So, we followed Obatala from his love of coconuts, to cocoa butter and didn't even mention another of his favorites – eggs. Well, Ayido Wedo also loves eggs so we will stop in with her next. She too, has a wide range of wisdom to share.

Ayido Wedo is one of my favorite *lwas*. She is the wife of *Dambullah*, and a celebrated snake deity of the Rada Vodou pantheon. Together, *Dambullah* and Ayido Wedo represent the powers of the sky. Ayido Wedo is very significant to the work in these pages. She symbolizes the rainbow, a bold synthesis of every different color. She is inclusive and considered a metaphorical representation of holism and integration. I see her as a symbol for integration of the mind, body, and spirit, which we are seeking in this weight-loss journey.

Together, Ayido Wedo, along with Dambullah, wrap their serpentine bodies around the world, and create; bringing life from thought to have form. I relate to the peaceful and tranquil nature of Ayido Wedo and use hers, as my magickal name. You may consult this *lwa* for bringing your thoughts into your form, and for, tranquility and blessings.

Ayido Wedo likes white foods, like Obatala. One of which is white eggs. Egg Magick is a cross-cultural phenomenon practiced in African traditions, the Baltic Region and by eclectic practitioners everywhere.

Things are to be tried, an old lady cooked stones and they produced soup.

Zimbabwean Proverb

Banish Evil and Protect Yourself with Cascarilla

Cascarilla (pronounced kas-kah-ree-ya) is made from pulverized egg shells. Egg shells hold life and creation within them, thus they are loaded with what is called in parts of Africa and the diaspora, *ashe*. *Ashe* is potentiality. Eggs are utilized in folk magic, such as my beloved Hoodoo, which we will delve into later.

Cascarilla is useful to your weight-loss plans because while slimming down, you are in a vulnerable state. You may meet with crushing criticism, indifference, negativity, enabling and other harmful influences. This powder made from white egg shells protects and banishes such influences.

Directions:

Either dry some white eggshells, completely and pulverize them to a fine powder with a mortar and pestle or purchase the blend premade at your local botanica. Use this power to conjure up the serene spirit of Ayido Wedo and the calm outlook of Obatala. This powder is also protective.

1. Banish evil influences, "haters" so to speak, from foiling your weight-loss progress with their own agendas.
2. Powder yourself with cascarilla.
3. Make a magickal ring of protection around your home, blocking out negativity, so you can undertake the serious work at hand.

Rastafari and I-tal

So far in this chapter we went into the healing potential and *ashe* of cayenne, coconut, cacao and eggs. What better place to go to deepen our understanding of the spiritual healing capabilities or *ashe* of certain foods than Jamaica?

Long before many of us even thought about eating organic or non-gmo (genetically modified foods), Rastafari celebrated these foods as a part of their spiritual outlook. Called I-tal, derived from the word "vital", with "I" replacing the "v" speaks to the interconnectedness of us all. Intense meditation and prayer of the type I am encouraging, is at the center of this form of spirituality, which calls Jamaica home. Rastafari beliefs are tracked all the way back to the 1930's, and is a Christian based movement with a deep connection to Ethiopia.

I mentioned I-tal because it is concerned with the life energy given by the higher power. For foods to have I-tal, they must be free of the following:

- Artificial sweeteners
- Artificial colors
- Preservatives
- Artificial flavors

In short, I-tal foods are the types of organic, non-gmo, whole foods you should be eating, right now. I-tal foods give 'livity'. Livity is the life energy given by God. I share the Rastafari predilection for I-tal, livity foods and their love for natural hair in the form of (dread) locks.

Now, you know already, we are not going to dwell on food. You need it to sustain yourselves. The higher quality the better. If you are taking this book seriously, you should be eating I-tal, livity foods, which are whole, organic, unpackaged or canned and non-gmo.

Jamaican Healing

Back in Section I. of this book, we discussed bush tucker also called wild foods. In Jamaica, there are also bush doctors who share their knowledge of wild foods. Bush doctors practice holistic health, with a focus on the mind, body, spirit connection to healing.

Maroons of St. Elizabeth Parish

There are some fascinating healers in Jamaica, and they have just the right medicinal plants and African-based wisdom to offer hope. There are called Mothers, healers that are also herbalists, catering to Moms-to-be. There are also Maroon healers. These healers are descendants of enslaved people, who revolted, ran away and won their freedom from slavery through their defiance and bravery. They intermarried with the indigenous Arawak people and live mostly in rural communities in the mountains. The maroons stand apart, having their own communities and celebrations. Dancing, singing, drumming and preparing traditions foods, the hallmark also for healing in this book, form the foundation of their healing ways.

Happiness is as good as food.

Maasai Proverb

Sexual Healing and Sexual Magick

Living close to the sea, in a tropical environment, with lots of warm nights and great music, makes Jamaica a sensual place. The healers in Jamaica have a lesson for us in the form of an aphrodisiac. Wait – but this is a weight-loss guide, why the inclusion of sex you might ask?

1. Good sex, three to five times per week can help you lose weight.
2. ½ hour of sex burns between 150–200 calories.
3. Sex enhances your mood by releasing chemicals in the brain called endorphins.
4. Sex can help you feel better about yourself.

Irish moss Drink

Jamaican healers that are Maroons, Bush Doctors and alternative health practitioners, recommend an ocean-inspired aphrodisiac mainly for men, called Irish moss drink. Irish moss (*Chondrus crispus*) is a type of seaweed, whose use was brought to Jamaica by early Irish immigrants. It is known the world over as a healthy tonic and good luck charm – both things we need for this work we've undertaken. The combination of ingredients in the drink also help with further issues we may encounter: indigestion, slow metabolism, anxiety, depression, and energy. Irish moss drink is a potion you can rest assured is loaded with vitamins and minerals.

Ingredients

¾ pound Irish moss

3 ounces ground gum Arabic

¾ cup honey

¾ cup maple syrup

5-ounces isinglass (a type of gelatin)

5-ounces of linseed[3] ground finely

3 tablespoons vanilla extract

5-quarts water

2 tablespoons powdered nutmeg[4]

1. Wash Irish moss to remove sand and grit from the ocean.
2. Rehydrate moss by putting it in water over night. Use 1 part of the moss to 2 parts water.
3. Place water in a pot; bring to a boil. Add Irish moss, gum Arabic, isinglass and linseed to the water.
4. Cook 45 minutes and you'll notice everything except the Irish moss will dissolve.
5. Strain, reserving the liquid.
6. Add the sweeteners, extract and nutmeg.
7. Simmer on low heat 10 minutes covered; cool thoroughly on the stove top.
8. Refrigerate for 6 hours or more. Serve chilled, in a shot glass and enjoy what comes next!

---

3 Also called flaxseeds
4 If you grate your own nutmeg it will lend an excellent flavor profile to the drink.

Sinkle Bible: Jamaican Cure-all

Another highly-touted drink and herbal medicine is Aloe Vera which is called Sinkle Bible by Jamaicans. Aloe can be used judiciously, not to excess. It helps with regularity when you are suffering from either diarrhea or constipation. It cleanses and purifies the colon, inspiring what could be a sluggish digestion system and making it more receptive to releasing weight.

Sinkle Bible is TLC (tender loving care) for your guts and belly by doing all of this:

- Cleansing the kidney, bladder, stomach and intestines
- Acting as a bitter
- Dealing with correcting imbalances
- Breeding good bacteria in the gut

To use: (here is a chance to put all your studies and things you've learned about African diaspora healing to work)

1. Select a leaf that calls to you; thank the leaf for sharing its medicine with you.
2. Wash it and pat dry.
3. Slit the leaf open while appreciating that it is giving you its medicine.
4. Saying your favorite prayer.
5. Put the juice from the leaf in a glass and drink it.

Motherland Herbalism: What's in it for you?

This chapter has been grounded in African Healing Ways. To bring together the wisdom shared in this chapter we must go to the Motherland. First understand an overview of the terminology used in its healing. Then, we will close with ways you can use the terms and concepts for your weight-loss journey:

Ashe

Organic objects are naturally imbued with potentiality and healing *ashe*, so they have a universal energy force within, connecting us all like an umbilical cord. Medicines, whether designed to address spiritual or physical complaints, are believed to derive their power from *ashe*.

Ashe is present in nature, herbal products and art and craft made from nature materials. The herbal teas, incense powders, spiritual washes, healing balms, charms, medicine bundles and even the purposefully spoken word, you are working with in this book, all contain *ashe*.

Good words are food;
bad words poison.

Malagasy Proverb

Ase

A West African word translates roughly to "spiritual blessings," *Ase* is a term for when an illness is addressed directly in its own language. Another meaning is the use of powerful herbs which are chewed ritualistically as the power words called *"ase*-words" are spoken.

ASE WORDS and TALK FIRE OUT OF BURNS

This *ase*-word practice knows no borders. It manifests in many forms in the diaspora. Here is a curious tradition that has been recorded on the coastal plains of North Carolina, wherein ailments like burns are talked right out of the body. The practice appropriately called, *"talk fire out of burns"* utilizes incantations.

The incantations almost always invoke angels. Here is one:

There came two angels from the north
One brought fire; and one brought frost
Go out fire and come in frost.[1]

The American, **Talk Fire out of Burns** practice stems from the same type of direct communication and understanding of the root ailment that is utilized in West Africa. You can work with this practice to talk your body into releasing its excess weight.

---

1 Thomas Stroup, "A Charm from North Carolina and The Merchant of Venice, II, vii, 75." *Journal of American Folklore*, 49 (1936), 266.

Daliluw

Daliluw are the recipes and techniques for mixing the various medicinal constituents. Herbal chemistry is used but some *daliluw* require spoken healing words also called *ase* words and other metaphysical rituals during preparation.

Bringing Spirit Home

Organic objects are replete with potentiality and healing *ashe*. They have a universal energy force within, connecting us all like an umbilical cord.

It is important to address each element or aspect of nature with the assertion that it is alive and our partner. This approach puts us in touch with the past, present, ancestors, nature spirits at once. Knowing we share stewardship with a living world, we do not own but are a component of, allows us to move easier towards a spiritually-rich, sustainable future. Borrowing practices from the complex realm of African spirituality helps build new traditions and spiritual practices that put us in touch with the spirit realm enriching our soul and facilitating releasing your weight.

Got Your Mojo Workin'?

Recently, I saw a documentary on YouTube, filmed 1961–1965 of Blues Men. Within it, there is a remarkable performance of the young Muddy Waters, he sings of getting' his mojo workin'. While watching, I asked the people around me if they knew what he was singing about. No one had a clue.

Mojo bags have incredible power and they can help with you are trying to do. I have done copious research into mojo bags and have tracked their development here in the United States back to the Motherland. This is only an abbreviated version of my studies in that area. If you want to know more, refer to my books dedicated to Hoodoo, "Sticks, Stones, Roots and Bones," and "365 Days of Hoodoo."

Central African Medicine Bags

Mojo bags are unmistakably a type of American medicine bag with an African influence. Medicine bags are a collection of power objects contained in a pouch or bag. In Central Africa, they are charged through feeding an infinite variety of natural materials, though some are manmade, including glass and gun powder. The best examples of these magical figures or accumulative sculptures come from Central Africa. The Yaka, Suku and Kongo peoples prepare sachets made from either: shells, baskets, pots, bottles or food tins, plastic bags or leather bags. In the west, this type of practice is considered 'sympathetic magick'.

Medicine Bags: from Africa to the New World

The Bamana of the Western Sudan use power objects such as medicine bags that are imbued with *ashe* for addressing various ills. These objects are used to express power as warriors, to fight supernatural malaise and to foil evil intentions. The bags contain *bilongo* (medicine) and a *mooyo* (a soul).

Soul Bags

One can well imagine enslaved Congo and Angolan medicine people bringing the concept of *bilongo* and *mooyo* together in the New World, to produce what we call *mojo bags*. In addition to the conceptual connection of *mooyo* as soul [bag], there is the visual connection between the words *mooyo* and mojo, which may suggest it is an Anglicized translation.

In Hoodoo practice, Mojo bags are prepared by a specialist called a hoodoo, two-headed doctor, rootworker or conjurer. With the aid of their soul food, the individual objects within each bag become an accumulative force that guides the spirits to understand the reason their help is sought.

Minkisi/Nkisi

So far, in our work in this book we have always considered nature as the heart of spiritual practice for aid in weight-loss. Within this work we consider gods, goddesses, supernatural being, and spirits, and their connection to the elements.

Kongo power figures are called *minkisi* or *nkisi* plural. *Nkisi* include elemental objects for example representative of land, sky, fire and water. *Nkisi,* also called charms, are empowered by the spirit of nature. These figures help people heal. They can serve as a safe spot or hiding place for the soul. They might contain sea shells, feathers, nuts, berries, stones, bones, leaves, roots or twigs.

Nkisi are as diverse and plentiful as the types of illnesses that exist on earth for example:

Nkisi Figures

In another form of empowering feeding, the Yaka, Kongo, Teke, Suku and Songhai pack a cavity in the belly of their sculptures with a wide array of *ashe*-containing materials: bones, fur, claws, elephant foot prints; crocodile teeth, scales and sexual organs' lightning excreta; bones, flesh and nails of sorcerers; remnants of suicide victims and of warriors. The figurines are then covered with the skins of power animals: buffalo, wild cats, lizards, antelope and birds, and they are then decorated with raffia, cloth, bells, beads, metal and nails.

Other materials encased in a mojo bag include ephemera associated with the dead: coffin nails, ground bones or graveyard dirt. The objects, whether stick, stone, root or bone have a corresponding spirit (ancestral, deity or natural) and the medicinal language ascribed to it.

Herbal Spirit Doll

Now that you've read all this, you probably want to make it real and practical, integrating some of its elements into your work. We can do that by incorporating some aspects of these concepts of viewing the world of African healing into your life and your spiritual journey toward weight-loss.

Reviewing the terms and types of spiritual objects you just read about, I want you to use some of the *ashe*-contained materials mentioned, to make a spirit doll representing your healthy new self. This doll is a manifestation of how you will be by the time you meet your goals.

Have you ever thought about what it would be like if your spiritual being and soul could take on a physical form? What would it look like, smell of, feel like or consist of? I would like you to set aside some time, it might not be today, but sometime soon. This time is set aside for you to get in touch with the sensory aspects of transformed self after you have met your weight-loss goals.

Begin the process with journaling and meditation to get in touch with your authentic self.

Look at the Check-in Sheet from Section I. of the book to think of spirits, gods or goddesses' qualities you would like to add to your spirit doll.

Use a self-selected combination of fabric, twigs, fibers, buttons and beads to create the outside of the Herbal Spirit Doll. Inside you will place symbolic bones and organs created from a variety of roots, pods, berries, leaves, buds, moss and bark collected from outside your home. Add your choice of fabric scraps, favorite buttons, and recycled materials, dried herbs from your garden, special beads, twigs, sea glass and stones to enhance the unique qualities of your spirit doll as you work. Afterwards, spray her with a suitable combination of the essential oil blends given in from Chapter 3 or healing flower water from Chapter 4. I hope you finish your doll before moving to the next chapter. You need her with you.

If you are of African descent, even if you don't know the names of some of these practices, they may be strangely familiar to you, something you know about in your bones or that you've observed in the workings of elder healers. Whatever your heritage, there are important lessons within the practices, traditions and spirituality of Africa and the diaspora. I hope this wisdom will ease your passage as you go about your weight-loss journey.

Speaking of journeying, we travel next to Asia, to see what we can learn from the impressive corpus of wisdom contained in Indian medicine.

CHAPTER 6

Shakti: Noticing, Acknowledging and Balancing

Ganesha the Gatekeeper

In Chapter 5, we entered the gates to African Healing Ways through the Legbas. Every pantheon and path has a gatekeeper. This is the deity or spirit you consult before beginning your work. We are moving into Indian healing now and we shall enter through the graces of Ganesha. Hindu god Ganesha, is the door opener and gate keeper to our work which follows.

We need Ganesha, at this point in the journey because he is both Lord of Success and destroyer of obstacles. Having stuck with this book and your weight-loss journey up to this point, Ganesha is the god you want in your corner when things get rough. He is celebrated as the god of learning, wisdom and knowledge, recurring themes in this chapter.

I must admit, Ganesha is one of my favorites. How can one not love the Lord of Obstacles and New Beginnings? With his elephant-head and pot-bellied human body, Ganesha is worshiped by millions across the planet, including not only Hindus but Buddhists, neo-pagans and Jains. Lucky for all, he is known to share his gifts of good fortune with everyone who approaches him with an honest heart and the things that he likes. Like others mentioned in this book, you mustn't anger him or he will turn his goodwill against you, throwing obstacles in your way, instead of removing them.

Ganesha prefers fresh starts, innovation and new visions. He also admires changes, such as those you are making in your life. Ganesha holds court over portals, entryways, thresholds and the magical place called the crossroads. When you are engaging him, venerate him first, as we are here. He must be invoked at the inception of your work. From there, he will work with you to heal ills of the mind, body and spirit. Ganesha favors a wide range of people including artists, authors, poets, musicians and those that approach him with openness and sincerity.

Ganesha Altar

If you feel the call to have Ganesha as your door opener, remover of obstacles and vessel of knowledge, to begin your work make a special space to venerate him.

1. Get a statue that represents him. Try to get one that includes his animals, the snake and the mouse which he is sometimes riding.
2. Go to your nearest Indian neighborhood to buy some modaka, his favorite dessert.
3. Place a white, pink or red cloth beneath his statue.

4. Put the cake on the plate, along with other sweets like bananas and a piece of fresh sugar cane.

Keep this space fresh and well stocked. Go to Ganesha, when your journey is headed in a new direction or you need redirection. This could happen because you go off your eating and exercise plan and need to start again or because you reach a plateau. This is the place to go, when you've fallen off track and need to begin again. It is also where you can gain wisdom.

Lakshmi

Few engagements with the gods, goddesses, supernatural spirits and beings make me as happy and fulfilled as invoking Lakshmi. I gently coaxed her into my living room with soft candles, incense and flowers. She appeared, resplendent with all her breathtaking beauty.

Lakshmi of the Hindu pantheon can help you with the journey to which you've dedicated yourself. She extends her devotees beauty. If you stick with her, she will shower you with abundance and good fortune of all sorts. She is also playful in spirit, and sensual. Lakshmi has a penchant for pleasures. She is a seeker and provider of joy.

Lakshmi comes as a vision, at first, hard to make out. That is because she beams with bright light, even her skin glows. Lakshmi doesn't appear or stick around without your dedication. Like many of the gods and goddesses engaged in this book, who are from the realm of beauty, she can be a bit short on the old attention span, moving along, if not honored properly and on a regular basis, to the next bright shiny experience.

Lakshmi appreciates it when you are attentive to her image. Gaze at it with your full attention and a sense of openness. Fete her with marigold flowers, lotus incense and conch shells. I usually burn the lotus incense over the shell.

The beautiful and voluptuous goddess Lakshmi asks you to love yourself and to show off your curves as she does. She is also the embodiment of the very healthy, sacred plant called Tulsi, which we will explore next.

Basil (sacred or holy) "Tulsi" *(Ocimum sanctum)*

Lakshmi is the incarnation of Tusli, the healing herb. This is a place where aromatherapy and spirituality come together, opening new dimensions in pleasure, health and happiness. Like many people, I had a fixed perception of basil. In the west, we think of basil primarily as a culinary herb used in Italian cooking, a salad or perhaps a sandwich. In India, one species of basil is considered a sacred herb. The Latin word *basilicum* supports this Indian conception; *basilicum* translates roughly as royal or princely. In India, the herb is commonly called Tulsi. It is also referred to as Bhutagni (destroyer of demons) Tulsi is thought of as a divine incarnation of the goddess; worshippers of Vishnu perceive the plant as the goddess Lakshmi, devotees of Rama see Tulsi as Sita; Krishna bhaktas view the herb as Vrinda, Radha or Rukmani.

There are numerous legends, called pura-katha (ancient tale) or divya-katha (divine story) in India that revolve around sacred basil. In the divya-katha, "Churning of the Cosmic Ocean" Vishnu obtained Tulsi from the rough ocean waves as an aid to the health of all beings.

In Sanskrit, the sacred herb is regarded as an incarnation of Tulasi. Tulasi was the wife of a celestial being, blessed by Lord Krishna, so everyone could worship her. Offerings are not complete unless they include Tulasi's blessings. Many types of incense are named for these goddesses, graced with the names Tulsi, Tulasi, Lakshmi and Laxmi.

Healing Qualities of Tulsi

Use of Indian sacred herbs so intimately connected to deities, such as Tulsi, is greatly enhanced by a basic understanding of Ayurveda. The word Ayurveda is derived from the words "Ayu" (life) and "Veda" (science). The ancient concepts of Ayurveda continue to influence and direct the use of healing herbs and aromatic treatments. Ayurveda is rooted in cherished scriptures called Vedas that date back to 1500 BC. The Vedas are sacred literature including the Rig-Veda that contains 1,000 hymns, written from 1,700–800 BC. The Rig-Veda still assert influence on Indian healing traditions.

In Ayurvedic practice, the mind exerts profound influence on the body. A well-balanced, tranquil mind, can free the body from illness. Acute awareness is central to achieving the necessary balance required for healing. The elements; as well as nature, talisman, amulets and symbols each play an important role in Ayurvedic healing.

One of the most promising qualities of Tulsi, within this ancient Indian system of medicine is *Moksa-prade*. *Moksa-prade* substances keep the body healthy and our minds free from worry, enabling concentration on spirituality and inner peace. Inner peace is that missing piece that makes us feel lacking and empty, leading to over-eating.

Growing and Using Tulsi

Visit your home and garden center or order Tulsi from an online supplier. Tulsi thrives in the pleasant climate of India. In temperate zones, it can be grown from seed, beginning indoors during April in a moist, peaty soil. This herb is a vigorous grower, usually reaching 18″ high. It should be placed outdoors in mid-June in pots, window boxes or directly in the garden. Grow Tulsi outside your home or business, as a natural amulet to encourage blessings and as a protective plant. Pinching back the top of the plant insures healthy growth and prevents an unattractively tall, leggy appearance. Use pinched-clippings in culinary or magickal recipes.

Tulsi Bundles

A simple, fragrant and magickal use of tulsi is to create a natural amulet using a tied bundle of the herb. Take a few clippings (approximately 10–12″ long) from the plant, tie firmly with a green (for healing, love, and life) ribbon, in a bunch. Hang the tulsi bundle, upside down, away from direct sunlight or heat, in the home – especially the kitchen. Tulsi bundles attract prosperity but more important to you, it draws health and good spirits. These are ideal for hanging just before seeking a new direction on your weight-loss path.

Diwali Lakshmi Ritual

Diwali is a two-week long celebration in late October through mid-November (starting date varies). The Hindu people use

Diwali as a period to vanquish ignorance by driving away darkness that engulfs the light of knowledge. Diwali is a festival of lights; the word is derived from the Sanskrit word Deepavali "deepa" meaning light and "avali" meaning row. Set up hanging lamps or as many candles in a row as possible to encourage the presence of Diwali. Welcome Lakshmi to this festive celebration. Lakshmi is embodied in basil, rice, coins and other symbols of prosperity and fertility. To invoke the blessings of Lakshmi during Diwali infuse a cup basil leaves in 4 cups of water. Strain. Add 8 drops holy basil essential oil.

Henna: Last Night's Herbal Interlude

Lakshmi loves henna too and so do I. The night before I wrote this, I set aside some mental space and physical space, right in my living room to consort with her. With minimal fuss and no messiness, I applied mehendi to the palm and topside of my right hand. So, as I type these words, my right-hand sports a flourish of swirling abstract patterns. They travel from the top of my hand to fingertips and then to the other side, where it graces my palms. I can still smell the unmistakable aromatic treat of deep earthy cloves, bright and clean eucalyptus and sweet, delicate rose water. I want to share this experience, while it and its magick, are still fresh in my mind and on my writing hands.

History of Henna

Before we proceed, understanding a bit of henna's history is in order. It is important to respect this plant and the magical substance it yields. That is at the request of Lakshmi. She gets very upset if henna is not respected. Bear that in mind, if you decide to apply it to yourself to invoke her.

Henna is an herbaceous shrub called *Lawsonia inermis* in botanical Latin, named after the British explorer John Lawson in the early 1700s. The plant thrives in hot dry climates. Use of the herb is carbon dated back to 3,500 BCE and has had a continuing presence in human civilization recorded in the arts for 7,000 years.

Henna is a Persian word for a plant with many names. In India Hindus often call it *mehendi*, a name synonymous internationally with henna plant used for temporary tattoos.

Henna the Cool Medicine

Often in America we like the short cut – the bare bones because in our fast-paced world it helps us efficiently assimilate information. If we were to skim off the top of henna's surface in that manner, simply thinking it is one of two things: hair dye or temporary tattoo from a package we would be missing its gift to those needing healing energy from plants – the gift of Lakshmi's affectionate focus. A medicinal herb, henna has many potent and promising qualities such as being a source for divination and meditation. Its ritualistic use is employed during important rites of passage. It is also naturally cooling, soothing, and drying.

Henna is:

- Ayurvedic medicine, wherein, henna tea is taken to treat many ailments you may encounter during our work, including: headache, fever, and stomach pain.
- An aromatherapy scent derived from the fragrant henna flower, used to make *Gulhina* or *hina*. The oil can be applied neat (straight) dabbed on to the pulse points, temples or crown

of the head. The oil-based perfume called *Hina Mehndi* Attar or *Gulhina,* is a good aid to getting into the right mind frame to stay focused and on course with your transformation. It has a spicy, floral, musky scent, calming and balancing scents used by both men and women.

Henna Medicine for the Mind, Body and Spirit

One of the most revered qualities of henna is its ability to cool. You need to stay cool and steer the course to achieve your slimming goals. As you do so, it is a good idea to reflect on the cooling qualities of henna herb:

- The soothing patterns of *mehendi* tattoos are considered a calming influence that uplifts depression.
- Applying henna to the head cools down hot-headed thoughts which can overwhelm you, sabotaging your slimming; it also slows you down and helps restore balance while instilling relaxation and tranquility.
- Mehendi breeds patience; cultivates persistence and quells anxiety.
- Henna invites communal activity, as it is difficult to accomplish alone – best shared with family or friends who are either on your weight-loss journey with you or supportive of it.

Take my lead, as my mehendi fingers glide back and forth across the keyboard (wish you could see them). Allow henna the attribute of goddess Lakshmi, to imbue your life with its holistic health benefits, uplifting mind, body and balancing spirit with happiness, filling your heart and home with joy. Life is short. Henna forces us to slow down. Take some time with family or friends while enjoying the supreme desert healing medicine called by many names but what we know best as henna.

Sarasvati's Shakti

Shakti is translated from Sanskrit as power, force or energy. Hindu Goddess Sarasvati is Brahma's Shakti. Brahma is the father figure in Hindu's holy trinity. Sarasvati is beyond important to our work. She is the conduit between spirit and matter.

Sarasvati is the embodiment of intelligence. She is called 'power of knowledge' and has the ability of forming and helping us synthesize ideas, as well as, the deep concepts in Ayurvedic medicine, which we are going to be exploring shortly.

Sarasvati means essence (sara) of our self (swa).

Imagine this:

As you enter the stream of consciousness that leads to enlightenment and knowledge on your path to changing, Sarasvati is the flowing river facilitating your journey.

The flowing river of knowledge, known as Sarasvati will help you internalize the hymns and mantras shared in this chapter. Considered the Divine Mother, Sarasvati is Goddess of the Word. Close to all activities creative, she will pave our pathway, along the way we will be obtaining and utilizing the profound wisdom contained within Ayurveda medicine.

In the Rig Veda, Sarasvati is described in many ways, including being the "awakener of happy and noble thoughts." Closely aligned with poets, scribes, bards and presenters, Sarasvati's seed syllable or bija mantra is AIM, pronounced (ah-e em).

Her mantra for invocation and praise contains her seed syllable AIM.

Recite this to invoke her before reading the rest of this chapter:

Goddess Sarasvati Invocation Mantra

Om Aim Sarasvati Namaha
Pronounced in English like this:
Om ah-eem sar-as-vuh-tee na-ma-ha.

You are greeting the goddess, by saying "Om! Salutations to the Goddess Sarasvati." Keep offering to her on your desk including marigolds, lotuses or lotus oil, and sweet incense. This will encourage her presence while you are journaling about your weight-loss experiences.

Life Knowledge: The Art of Ayurveda

Prakruti (or the individual's constitution) is something you receive at the time of conception, as a fetus you have your own Prakruti and you inherit some from each of your parents. You will most likely die with the same Prakruti you were born with. On a cosmic level Prakruti is considered determined, active consciousness. It is the divine creative will. On a physical level, Prakruti is your body's individual combination of mental and physical traits. It is also your mind, body, spirit balance and consequently your ability to heal. The concept of Prakruiti refers to the general state of your health.

FINDING AN AYURVEDA PRACTITIONER

Ayurveda is widely practiced in contemporary India, Bangladesh, Sri Lanka, Nepal and Pakistan. 80% of the population in India for example, utilizes Ayurvedic medicine exclusively. In the United States roughly 200,000 people used some type of Ayurvedic treatment during the 2016.

I have included Ayurveda in this book because it is one of the ultimate forms of holistic, nature-based medicines dealing with the underlying issues of excess weight. In Ayurvedic Medicine it is believed that each person is an integrated part of the cosmos – each person embodies the universe. It is also believed that when we live in accord with the universe we will be healthy.

Within the Ayurvedic elaborate systems of medicine there is special attention paid to the root causes of obesity – primarily this issue arises from being out of balance with the universe. Before we return to the topic of obesity and how to treat it using Ayurvedic methods, first it is important to understand the basic concepts of this form of medicine.

Connection to the universe, the constitution of the body (Prakriti) and the life forces (doshas) are the founding principles in understanding and treating disease and instilling wellness.

Doshas (life forces) are three different energies with individual characteristics. Each dosha consists of two or more elements: ether, air, fire, water, earth. Doshas are in a constant state of flux changing with the wheel of the year, diet, and bodily functions. When doshas become unbalanced we become ill in ways specific to dosha makeup. Imbalance of dosha occurs from exposure to hazardous chemicals, germs and viruses and being subjected to harsh weather conditions. Imbalances may also be caused by the individual's age and life passage; lifestyle, diet and the level of physical or mental exertion or lack thereof.

Vata Dosha is dry, light, frigid, mobile, active, clear, crisp, astringent and a dispersing energy. Vata dosha individuals typically have a small body frame, lightly muscled, little fat, thin build, and can be underweight. Vata dosha has cold hands and feet, as well as poor circulation. They hate the cold and winter. Since they are very clear in perception, vata dosha is sometimes clairvoyant. Vata dosha's element is air

Pitta Dosha is hot, sharp, light, aqueous, sour, oily, spreading, strong smelling, represented by a sour or bitter taste. Pitta dosha individuals have a strong appetite, warm skin and body temperature that is higher than vata. If pitta doshas are hungry, they must eat right away otherwise they become angry, irritable and hypoglycemic. They have a sharply shaped-nose, teeth, eyes, mind, use sharp words, have a good memory, have oily, limp straight hair; oily bowel movements and are represented by liquid. Pitta's like to read books before bedtime and often fall asleep with the book. They lose their hair early and have the following chronic complaints: inflammatory disease, neurological muscular and rheumatic problems. Pitta dosha elements are fire and water.

Kapha Dosha is heavy, slow, cool, oily, liquid, dense, thick, stationary and cloudy. Kapha has a predilection for sweet and salty tastes. People with this dosha have big bones, large muscles and carry a lot of fat. Kapha dosha put on weight easily. The metabolism of kapha is slow; they walk and talk slowly. Kapha dosha has cold, damp skin, thick, wavy dark hair, big attractive brown eyes. This dosha has a slow but steady memory. Kapha people are forgiving, loving and compassionate with good endurance. They enjoy eating, staying stationary and not doing anything. Kapha dosha is aggravated by greed, napping, eating too many sweets, eating even though full as well as eating and drinking foods and beverages that are very salty or watery. Kapha are susceptible to diabetes, cancer, obesity, respiratory illness such as asthma and COPD. Most kapha's will find a need for this book to support their weight-loss journey.

RIDDING THE BODY OF TOXINS

Panchakarma (methods for ridding the body of ama) also called the five actions or five stepped practice, are an assortment of cleansing and purification methods prescribed by Ayurvedic doctors for certain diseases and for bi-annual cleansing.

The element of kapha is water and earth.

To determine dosha type an Ayurvedic doctor will ask you a series of questions about your family history, disposition, physical characteristics and environment. The doctor will also palpitate, take visual notes, and listen to your heart and lungs, and give you a thorough check up, carefully examining your tongue and eyes.

DON'T LET AMA FOIL YOUR WEIGHT-LOSS EFFORTS

Ama (waste; undigested food that stays in or on the internal organs and body tissue, leading to illness) is mind/body toxins, created by poor digestion and unhealthy lifestyle. Ama is accumulation that clogs the open conduits of the body and it breeds excess weight. There are several systems and herbs in Ayurveda to reduce or cleanse the body of ama.

Herbs to Reduce Ama in the Body

- Guggulu take with triphala
- Triphala
- Trikatu
- Barberry
- Turmeric

Ayurvedic Herbs for Weight-loss and Wellness

Ayurvedic Medicine utilizes herbs, metals, minerals or other materials. Currently there are over 600 ayurvedic herbal formulas and at least 250 single herbs used medicinally in the Ayurvedic pharmacy. In the next section, I will introduce a few of the key formulas and Ayurvedic herbs for weight-loss.

Triphala

Triphala is one of the most popular detoxification Ayurvedic formulas. The traditional supplement was first created thousands of years ago and is referenced in the early vedic texts of Caraka Samhita and Sushrut Samhita. The Caraka Samhita says it is as nourishing and useful as mother's milk. Triphala is considered the best, multipurpose herbal formula. It contains both nutritious and elimination qualities. Triphala nourishes the bones, reproductive organs and nervous system. All three fruits that it contains are proven antioxidants, therapeutic with wide and varied medicinal uses. Triphala is tridoshic rasayan; it balances and revitalizes all three doshas. This blend is valuable in the pursuit of weight-loss because it instills a healthy metabolism and reduces body wastes. It is prized as a panchakarma because it detoxifies and cleanses without being destructive or irritating to the colon.

Triphala means "three fruits." The three fruits used in triphala are amla, hataki and bibhitaki, each one corresponds to one of the three doshas. While best used in combination as Triphala, I am going to explain the benefits of each herb individually to give a better idea of the collective power of this healing formula.

Amla Botanical Description

Indian gooseberry, better known as Amla, is a renowned Ayurvedic and Unani medicine. Also called amalaki or dhartriphaia, (*Phyllanthus emblic, syn. Emblica officinalis)* is the botanical Latin name for Amla. Indian Gooseberry is a long living deciduous tree from the Euphorbiaceae family. All parts of the tree are used in Ayurvedic medicine including the root, bark, flowers, leaves, seed and fruit. Amla is well known both for its berry and the oil extracted from it which is commonly referred to as Amla. The two types of amla include gramya, the cultivated type and vanya, the wild type.

Amla's Indian History

Amla has an interesting history in India as a healer. It is called the nurse (Dhatri) and the sustainer (Amalaki). One of the reasons it is revered is because it contains five of the six rashas or tastes (bitter, pungent, sweet, astringent and sour) – the only taste it is missing is salty. This is important because a balanced meal should contain the six tastes to cultivate wellness and provide a grounded sense of satiety.

Amla is a natural ingredient good for the pitta dosha. The pitta dosha lives in the small intestine, stomach, sweat, blood, plasma and sebum. Amla is good for pitta dosha because it is cooling, while the natural inclination of a pitta dosha is to be hot.

The Phyto-Nutrients in Amla

Indian Gooseberry consists mostly of water – as much as 80%. It is a rich source of vitamin C, minerals such as iron; protein, carbohydrates and fiber. The vitamin C it contains is important because it is a necessary part of the synthesis of collagen. Amla fruit contains about 20 times more vitamin C than our usual source, the orange. Amla is rich in antioxidants and polyphenols.

Amla Cures

- Improves thinking capacity
- Detoxifies the system
- Rejuvenates body
- Boosts immunity
- Supports heart, liver, lung and bone health
- Balances stomach acids
- Improves mental instability

Herbal Actions

Amla is a tonic, rejuvenator, astringent, aphrodisiac, laxative, refrigerant and stomachic. Amla can be eaten or consumed as a drink or taken in capsule form as an internal treatment for all conditions mentioned.

Haritaki (Terminalia chebula)

Haritaki contains five of the six rashas, with a predominately bitter taste. The vata dosha, air and ether elements are correlated with haritaki. This herb treats imbalances and diseases of vata dosha.

Haritaki History

Haritaki is so revered by the Buddhists that the small fruit is painted in the hands of medicine Buddha in sacred paintings called tankas. Haritaki translates: one who came from Hari (God's) home. When Indra, King of the Hindu deities, was drinking the nectar of heaven a drop of it fell to earth introducing us to Haritaki. Haritaki contains all the rashas (tastes) accept salty. The herb is useful in so many ways that it is considered primary medicine. Haritaki is valuable in fighting obesity and being overweight. It stokes the digestive fires, making even the tiniest bits of nutrients readily absorbed by the body. It has the property of digesting the undigested. Haritaki contains the strongest laxative in the triphala formula.

Haritaki Plant Profile

The haritaki tree grows 50–80 feet at various altitudes. The tree grows in sub-Himalayan tracks from Ravi to West Bengal as well as in deciduous forests. The fruit is typically harvested during the spring.

Herbal Actions of Haritaki

Haritaki possesses laxative, astringent, lubricant, antispasmodic and nervine properties. It is used to treat severe and chronic constipation, nervous disorders like anxiety and stress, as well as combating a feeling of heaviness. This herb is rejuvenating and a versatile curative.

Curative Effects of Haritaki

- Heart tonic
- Promotes wisdom
- Antioxidant
- Laxative
- Paste of the fruit reduces swelling
- Treats gastrointestinal disorders
- Aids digestion
- Is an anti-inflammatory
- Prevents kidney stones
- Taken with honey it helps fight obesity
- Helps with weight-loss by aiding in smooth absorption of food
- Helps with Diabetes
- Treats hemorrhoids
- Deters skin disorders
- Prevents vomiting
- Stops hiccups
- Helps with liver and spleen health
- Prevents heart disease

Obesity and Haritaki

This herb is best taken by those at their goal weight or those who are overweight. It must be used sparingly if a vitiated pitta dosha condition is present.

Taken with rock salt, Haritaki addresses the aggravated Kapha dosha helping those that are overweight lose weight.

Bibhitaki (*Belleric myrobalan. E*)

The third fruit used in Triphala or "the three fruits." Bibhitaki is a specific treatment for Kapha dosha and helps break down fat in the body, reducing excess weight. This herb is astringent, bitter, sweet and warm; it affects the lungs, heart and liver. Bibhitaki contains 35% oil and 40% protein.

History

Bibhitaki means "the one who keeps you away from the diseases." The tree is *Vihhitaki* in Sanskrit which means fearless.

Bibhitaki Tree

Bibhitaki is a tall, deciduous tree with a buttressed trunk, brownish-grey bark with shallow lengthwise fissures. It can grow 60 to 80 feet. The parts used in Ayurvedic medicine are the fruits and bark. The fruits are oval, grey and contain an inner kernel. Bibhitaki is naturalized throughout the Indian subcontinent and grows in Sri Lanka and Southeast Asia up to 1,200 meters in a wide variety of biomes. It is also cultivated in large cities.

Weight-loss Herbal Actions of Bibhitaki

- Tonic
- Digestive
- Cardiovascular

Curative Actions of Bibhitaki for Weight-loss Issues

- Gas
- Hemorrhoids
- Headache

- Skin disorders
- Water weight gain
- Constipation
- Diarrhea

Green Tara

I can see a relationship between Green Tara (pronounced TAH-rah), the first woman to become a Buddha and the next herb we are going to discuss Guggulu. There are many Taras. Green Tara is a healing Tara.

Green Tara's left hand has blue lotuses, which represent power and purity. In her right hand, you will find that she has taken on the refuge and grant-making posture, called a mudra. As a Buddha of action, she is poised and ready to stand up, acting as your savior if need be.

She brings us towards enlightenment and spiritual wisdom. Green Tara eliminates suffering much in the same way as Guggulu, the herb. You may be feeling fear or anxiety from time to time. You will wonder if your efforts are worth it when temptation strikes. Another question that arises is whether you will meet your goal or will this transformation change your relationship to family and friends? It will most definitely change your relationship to food. For many, changes that are as substantial as the ones you might be encountering cause fear and anxiety. Green Tara can help you maneuver the choppy waters you will encounter, by helping you navigate challenging situations that arise. That is why I want you to sing or recite this hymn to invoke Green Tara when you encounter fear or anxiety. This hymn celebrates her attributes, as witnessed in her iconography:

On a lotus seat, standing for realization of voidness,
(You are) the emerald-colored, one-faced, two-armed Lady
In youth's full bloom, right leg out, left drawn in,
Showing the union of wisdom and art - homage to you!

Like the outstretched branch of the heavenly turquoise tree,
Your supple right hand makes the boon- granting gesture,
Inviting the wise to a feast of supreme accomplishments,
As if to an entertainment-homage to you!

Your left hand gives us refuge, showing the Three Jewels;
It says, "You people who see a hundred dangers,
Don't be frightened-I shall swiftly save you!"
Homage to you!

Both hands signal with blue utpala flowers,
"Samsaric beings! Cling not to worldly pleasures.
Enter the great city of liberation!"
Flower-goads prodding us to effort-homage to you!

First Dalai Lama 1391–1474

Guggulu

Guggulu is Sanskrit for "that which protects from diseases." This is an especially good herbal treatment for you because it is a weight-loss herb. Guggulu searches out and removes excess fat and toxins from the body. In addition to being a digestive aid and its uses in weight management Guggulu, the resin from the small, thorny mukul myrrh tree (*commiphora mukul*), improves strength, increases libido, reduces cholesterol, treats hemorrhoids, arthritis, soothes the nervous system and urinary system, quells skin disorders, and it revitalizes. Guggulu is soluble in water.

Agni – Digestive Fire

Agni is an Ayurvedic term that describes the digestive fire and is the name of the god of fire. Having Agni means that you can transform matter, like food, beverages, things you see, hear, smell, touch and taste and information, into yourself. Agni is about integration and assimilation of various parts. Balanced Agni also empowers you to properly digest food, making nutrients available to the body. Agni detoxifies the body's toxins removing excess waste. Through Agni, the body can become trim and fit, balanced and healthy. When someone is too low in Agni or high in Agni problems such as these arise:

Low Agni (a typical Kapha condition)
- Flatulence
- Indigestion
- Mental exhaustion
- Unfocused/dazed
- Light if any perspiration
- Dull complexion
- Obesity

High Agni
- Burping
- Heavy perspiration

- Skin eruptions
- Diarrhea
- Hyper-active
- Chatty
- Heart Burn
- Irritable
- Angry

Correcting Imbalanced Agni

- Take 4–5 small meals per day
- Drink citrus flavored water (squeeze lemon or lime slice into glass of water) throughout the day
- Drink warm ginger tea with honey
- Take trikatu before meals (see side bar)
- Sip boiled water with meals
- Eat pungent spices (especially Kapha dosha) like cumin, fennel and cardamom
- Build up saliva in your mouth to aid digestion
- Make sure right nostril is unobstructed to aid digestion

TRIKATU

Trikatu: ginger, black pepper and cayenne mixed; spread a pinch of this mixture over ¼ teaspoon of honey. Take before each meal.

EXERCISE FOR BALANCING AGNI

Put hands over navel. Close your eyes. Ground and center yourself.
Concentrate solely on your breathing. Notice hands moving up and down
on your belly with each breath. Now repeat this process but with this round
imagine a candle flame or the fire in a fireplace burning behind your navel.
Say the mantra:

Om Hum Agniye Namaha (om hoom agn-eye-yaye nama-ha)
I am the fragrance of the earth.

Lord Krishna

India's Sensual Fragrances

Intoxicating and delightful on their own, Indian herbs have been
processed for thousands of years, yielding some of the world's
finest perfumes and incenses. This is mind and spirit medicine.
In Ayurvedic practice, the mind exerts profound influence on the
body. You can lose weight when your mind is in a good place. Acute
awareness is central to achieving the necessary balance required for
healing. Stones, flowers, water, trees, herbs, talisman, amulets and
symbols each play an important role in Ayurvedic healing.

Aroma, released by fire or captured in oils is a key component
as well. As I write this segment, I have dabbed my chakras with
my favorite Indian ruhs and essential oils. There is a sandalwood
candle burning fragrantly on my desk and wafts of Nag Champa
billow softly overhead. If possible, join me in this aromatic journey
experience by lighting a dhoop (incense) stick or creating a dhoona
(sacred fire) using candles.

Fragrant Blessings from India

In India, there is an array of delightful scents, used for cleansing, health, beauty, ritual, prayer and magic. Here is a terminology key and usage notes for a few my favorite Indian fragrances.[5]

Attar: essential oils of often-precious flowers or herbs, obtained through hydro distillation. In India, attars are often extracted into a sandalwood base.

Otto: plant material that undergoes a similar process to attars; rose otto is one of the most widely used.

Ruh: Prepared in the same manner as attars but without the inclusion of sandalwood. Ruhs are extracted essences of precious flowers in concentrated form.

Gulhina *(Lawsonia inermis)*
This is perfume oil created from what is commonly called the henna plant. The flowers, called hina and the leaves, have been used as a refrigerant, cooling people for centuries in the hot climates of India. Hina is also astringent; helps treat headache, fever, insect bites, and painful joints. The oil-based perfume has a spicy, floral, musky scent. Mostly men wear Gulhina. Key to your ongoing progress and support system, it is also used in worship and ceremony.

---

5 Other Indian fragrances are in Section III. of this book.

Hina, Lord Shiva and Parvati

The symbolic power of hina rises from its association with Lord Shiva and Parvati his consort. Lord Shiva is the most powerful of all deities and he is the god of destruction. Parvati, decorated herself with henna to please him and win over his affections. Lord Shiva responded favorably to her charms, ever since then the herb is associated with sensuality. Since Shiva is a feared god, hina is also associated with protection of women. The herb is associated with rites of passage such as what we are going through.

Jasmine *(Jasminum officinale)*
Jasmine has an intensely sweet, almost narcotic perfume with hints of honey, fruit and green undertones. The sweet, romantic scent eases anxiety and aids sleep. To treat yourself for meeting your goals, maintaining or losing weight, try a jasmine hair accessory. It can be worn fresh, pinned to the hair. Motia is the Indian name for Jasmine attar.

TIP

To use motia, apply neat to pulse points (use sparingly).

Kewda *(Pandanus odoratissimus)*
Kewda is a superb mind, body, spirit medicine with a mysterious, penetrating scent. The top note is reminiscent of hyacinth yet it quickly fades to a gentle, rejuvenating scent.

TIP

Apply a dab of kewda attar neat, to chakras or pulse points.

Lotus *(Melumbo nucifera)*

In Hindu faith, the lotus, particularly the pink flower, is associated with Lakshmi. In art, Lakshmi is often featured standing on, or holding, lotus pods. Buddhists associate the lotus with purity, since neither the leaves nor the petals show traces of the mud from which it grows. Mythology around the plant grows from the fact that the stem and roots vanish beneath muddy water, while its delicate blossoms open towards the sky.

The white lotus, *(Nymphaea lotus L.,)* only blooms at night. The lotus symbolizes the awakening of the soul, as it reaches towards enlightenment and moves away from ignorance. Across the globe, the lotus symbolizes the duality of nature, as it exists in two realms, above and beneath the ground. It is a symbol of grace, beauty, women, opportunity and sensuality. The lotus also symbolizes the bounty and abundance of Green Tara and Laksmi, among others. Wearing the oil, a Mehndi tattooed image or amulet, sparks creativity and self-acceptance.

The scent is moist and watery, suggestive of the fecundity of the Great Earth Mother. Lotus oil comes from blue, white and pink flowers – each has a distinctive scent, blue or white are great for an introduction to lotus. The plant is slightly narcotic, causing sedation and deep relaxation. The lotus is believed to have been a gift from Egypt to India. The type commonly available today is *Nymphaea lotus.*

TIP

Apply pure lotus oil neat to pulse points or chakras for grounding and centering or to enhance sexuality.

Mitti (Baked Earth Attar)

Mitti is distilled earth, with an exquisite, rich, deep, mysterious smell. The perfumers of Kannauj gather the earth from dried lakes, ponds or wells for their fine earth aroma. They collect the caked earth and moisten it, then form dough and make coarse vessels which are then baked in handmade kilns with straw. When half-baked the vessels are moistened and then the lengthy distillery process begins. The scent derived from rain-soaked earth during the monsoon. The smell is evocative physically, spiritually and metaphorically, to all who encounter it.

Ruh Khus *(Vetiveria ziazaniodes)*

Ruh Khus also called the "Oil of Tranquility" is created from distilled wild-crafted vetiver grass, grown in Uttar Pradesh, Haryana, Madhya Pradesh and Rajasthan. Ruh Khus has fixative or scent preserving qualities in botanical blends and perfumes. It is a natural refrigerant, useful in cooling fevers or returning to balance after a passionate interlude. Ruh Khus is excellent perfumed oil, used neat, applied to pulse points or chakras. The oil cools the body during hot, steamy summer months.

To wear Ruh Khus, is to be enveloped in the sweet embrace of the Earth Mama, in her numerous incarnations. The smell suggests, earth, roots, dampness and it sparks creativity, fecundity, inspiration and fertility. Ruh Khus is an excellent scent for striking balance in our chaotic world and for bringing us into the inner sanctum of creation.

Sandalwood *(Santalum album)*

Sandalwood is beloved in numerous cultures as an aid to meditation, aphrodisiac, emollient, anti-inflammatory, mild astringent and for its ability to break insomnia.

The mellow scent of sandalwood eases inhibitions, builds self-confidence, induces a calm sedate mood, can assist in achieving a meditative state.

Incense enjoys a central role in Hindu faith. According to Hindu religious writing, worship must include burning fires of fragrant woods at the four cardinal points, where consecrated oils are placed. Sandalwood embodies the profound relationship between fragrance and spirituality in India and elsewhere.

Ayurveda: Your Prescription for Healing and Weight-loss

This chapter on Ayurvedic medicine focused specifically around its cadre of healing herbs. A key component to any weight-loss plan is exercise. The exercises suggested by Ayurvedic practitioners include increased safe sexual activity, walking at least 30 minutes a day, yoga and the mind/spirit exercise meditation. We will explore these types of exercise later. Massage is also an integral part of the Ayurvedic prescription for weight-loss. Contact your Ayurvedic practitioner for the appropriate massage as you embark on an Ayurveda diet and exercise plan.

Section II: Check-in

Once again it's time to take stock. As with your first assessment, you can copy and print this or jot down the questions and your answers in your personal journal. Either way it is now time for a brief break to check-in and spend time with self-reflection.

1. Did you lose any weight while working through this section?
2. How much weight did you want to lose?
3. How much did you actually lose?
4. Which of the stories about African or Asian cultures resonated the most with you and why?

_____

_____

_____

_____

_____

_____

5. There are many gods, goddesses and spirits explored in this dense section of the book. Which of these beings made the biggest impact on your lightening up loss journey?

_____

_____

_____

6. Of all the gods, goddesses and spirits explored, which of them inspired you the most?

_____

Why? _____

_____

_____

7. Did you do any of the recipes, altars, projects, affirmations or incantations?
   Of all the work you did, whether recipes, altars, projects, invocations, affirmations, meditation or incantations, which helped you with your health journey the most and why?

_____

_____

_____

_____

_____

_____

_____

Part III

Completing the Circle

CHAPTER 7

Elemental Rites of Passage

As *Earth Mama's Spiritual Guide to Weight-loss* circle draws near a close, there is still one last bit of important ground to cover. This section, apart from your reflections at the end of section I and II, might be the most important part of the books' work. This final chapter encourages you to embrace your new-self, with the help of the elements, herbs, friends, family, ceremony and ritual.

Elemental Magick

Every Earth Mama, and Papa too for that matter, are surrounded by, and hopefully engaged in the elements of earth, air, water, fire and ether; which makes their acknowledgement and use the most natural way to close the circle the book creates, though your weight-loss journey is likely to be life-long.

Embrace the Changes

One of the most challenging aspects of the weight-loss journey for me isn't losing the weight, it is embracing myself after the weight has come off, and maintaining. After taking off 50 pounds, I asked myself: who is this new person I see passing the mirror or window, when it should be me? Much of the human brain is programmed to identify faces: whose face was that in the mirror, in place of mine?

After a while, you get use to yourself but when a drastic change is made, be it short haircut, piercing, tattoo or weight-loss, you find that this change catches your eye. You remember how things were; longer hair, plain skin or a larger body. Obviously, you've invited the change, initiated it and potentially paid for it (depending on the change) that doesn't guarantee that you embrace it, welcome it, or will keep it.

To my mind, one of the primary reasons we snap back, and put on weight or return to how we were, is because we reject the change. We don't like to change, yet for health or other reasons, it becomes necessary.

Belly Wisdom

People that are naturally thin and don't struggle with their weight, don't get this journey from their gut. When I'm seeing a rail thin dietician or nutritionist, who is in her 20's, I wonder, how could he or she possibly get this? How would this person (or anyone else) know the full complexities of my weight-loss struggle well enough to be truly helpful?

Indeed, one of the reasons many of us shy away from seeing such people is because we intuit they think we are in a state of mystery…we don't understand how to eat, how much to exercise… how to maintain. They also assume we're miserable. Sometimes we are. Sometimes we aren't. And, yes, there is an element of mystery or misery, but there is also a leeriness of the entire process and of opening it all up to outsiders who might not get it. Those of us in the struggle, get it from the head and gut's many intelligences.

Before continuing, I must say, many heavier-bodied people are very knowledgeable of how to eat, sometimes more so than their thinner counterparts, but we make alternate choices. Most of us have little problem with the knowingness, it is with the ability to embrace and sustain life changes.

So, I acknowledge this leery feeling. You may feel it while reading this book, but trust me – I know the battle. I've lived it for my entire adult life, and it is not over. It is an on-going process. I want to inspire and show some interesting tips but I don't claim to know all the answers. It took me about 14 years to write this book, and I keep re-reading it to try to really "get" the essence of it, on a gut level.

Sustainable Weight-loss

Anyway, how do we go about accepting changes to our shape? To be successful, we need to not only be accepting, we must be willing to maintain the weight-loss through a daily, weekly, monthly and yearly regimen. Now, these changes might be 10, 15, or 100 pounds. People in each group struggle with maintenance – what I call sustainable weight-loss.

The answer, is through spirituality. Work your spirituality, connect to the Earth Mama and stay busy working on either reaching or maintaining what you've worked so hard to accomplish (or want to accomplish). Weight-loss is very hard work!

But for now, let's delve into playful ways we can embrace ourselves utilizing the Earth Mama as a vehicle.

Earth: Embracing the Changes

Earth Mama as a goddess is verdant, grounding, supportive, nurturing, facile and comforting. This exercise is simple to do and can be done indoors or out. I'm hoping you can embrace every element of Earth Mama, as you work.

Sand Drawing

If you can go to the beach, of a lake, pond, or sea, to undertake this ritual, you're in luck. You have freedom of practically endless proportions.

Secondly, you can go to a sandbox. You may have one outside your home or a local one, where you'd feel comfortable.

For other's, a portable indoor sandbox or sand table might just do the trick.

Sand Drawing is meditative. It also reconnects you to your inner-child, which is the very spot where some of your addiction, if you have one, may have started. The work you will do is ephemeral – temporary and transient. It lends itself to being non-judgmental by the very nature of its impermanent quality.

The work is to get in touch with your spirits. Did you happen to connect with any of the deities, lwa or orisha we explored? Perhaps you want to just get in touch with your inner-child by scribbling. To do any of this, you will need to get into a very relaxed and open state. I suggest:

1. Meditating for 15–20 minutes
2. Practicing pranayama, where your breathing is important to

your movement. This is especially well-suited to beach work.

3. A spiritual wash to get in touch with deity, lwa or orisha, made into a ritual by employing their favorite incense and essential oils related to them.

Once you are most relaxed, with a clear head, and limber body, you are ready.

MAKING A MOBILE SANDBOX

Sandboxes are used indoors and out. Sand is used on tables and for indoor Japanese gardening.

1. Buy high quality play sand from a garden center or lumber yard. You can also scoop some up from the beach and take it home.
2. Grab a container. So many different types will work. A plastic container with a lid that is about a foot and a half deep, is ideal.
3. Pour about a foot of sand into the box.

Now, we're ready to work. This type of work takes best under the New Moon. You will need a small container of water and some drawing tools. Your hands are fine, or you can use a combination of: a small rake, whisk broom, spoon, fork, blunt knife, palette knife, stick, paint brush handle and/ or pencil.

MOON and MAGIC

We can accomplish a great deal under the natural light of the sun. There's still more to do under the light of the moon. There are many complexities to Moon Magic, and whole books have been written about it. Briefly, in Wicca, for beginner and intermediate practice, the New Moon is for beginning and developing new projects or spiritual work; Full Moon is for adding a blast of full power to your work; Waning to Dark Moon, is for getting rid of things and banishing them.

Preparing for Elemental Healing Ritual

I have just discussed sandalwood in the previous chapter, but want to go into greater detail here, into the ways you can use it now to prepare for your final rituals and ceremonies, in relation to the elements.

Mailaagar bereh hai bhuyiangaa. Bikh amrit basahi ik sangaa.
The snakes encircle the sandalwood trees. Poison and nectar dwell there together.

The Divine Teachings of Gurbani (Sri Guru Granth Sahib, SGGS 525)

In India, the heartwood of sandal trees, from which sandalwood is derived, has divine status. It is a manifestation of divinity and holiness. The oil is used to anoint images of sacred deities, because it is considered pleasing to the gods. Sandalwood is used in the last rites of Hindus; the wood is used on funeral pyres to carry the soul to its eternal abode.

Sandalwood is beloved in numerous cultures as a spiritual aid to meditation and devotion. Medicinally, it is cooling, aphrodisiac, emollient, anti-inflammatory and mildly astringent. Sandalwood is also admired for its ability to break insomnia. The psychological (aromachology) applications of sandalwood include easing inhibitions, boosting self-confidence, inducing a calm sedate mood, as well as releasing emotions.

Sandalwood and the Elements

Air

Sandalwood essential oil is the concentrated extract of the heartwood of the sandal tree. The oil is considered an aphrodisiac that builds self-confidence and generates wellness in the workplace or living environment. Sandalwood essential oil is widely available and works well dispersed by air by doing one of the following:

- Add appropriate amount to an aromatherapy-vaporizing unit.
- Light a votive candle beneath the unit. (Never leave this unattended)
- Add oil to a scent ring that works with a regular light bulb. Follow manufacturer's directions.

Water

To release sandalwood energy in water, try one of the following:

- Add pure sandalwood hydrosol to a spray-top bottle; spray face and hair for conditioning, spiritual benefits and balancing of moods.
- During rinsing of hand washables, add ½ cup sandalwood hydrosol to wash basin. Swirl fine linens, lingerie or scarves in this water; complete process appropriate for the fabric, using clothing manufacturer's directions. Hang outdoors to dry, to magnify the power of the herb, if possible.
- Purchase readymade unscented bubble bath, shampoo, conditioner or lotion. Add suggested amount of sandalwood for quantity of product. Mix thoroughly before use.
- Create melt and pour (M & P) soap using the manufacturer's

directions. Scent opaque or clear glycerin M & P soap, with sandalwood essential oil.

Earth and Fire

- Apply neat (straight sandalwood essential oil) to the chakras or pulse points; body heat will disperse the scent. The oil is gentle enough to use on humans or animal companions.
- Sandalwood oil is used as a base for many fine herbal perfume oils from India called attars (attar, of the air and wind) including Gulhina from the *(Lawsonia inermis) plant;* Kewda *(Pandanus odoratissimus);* Motia *(Jasminum officinale)* and Rose *(Rosa damascena).* These are also applied neat to temples, pulse points or chakras.
- Sandalwood oil and the attars above can be used to massage yourself or receive massage; diluted with sweet almond oil or jojoba oil. Add ½ teaspoon to 8 ounces of oil; swirl to mix.
- Light an unscented candle for a few minutes. When there is a pool of melted wax extinguish candle. Add a couple drops sandalwood essential oil to candle and relight.

One of the most satisfying ways of combining sandalwood with fire, is the age-old practice of enjoying smoldering incense.

RECOMMENDED

- Baiedo (Japanese) Incense and ethically-harvested pure-grade sandalwood oil, if you decide to use essential oils.
- Engage in the delightful sandalwood tree, in whichever combination of elemental ways you choose, before moving on to the next ritual.

Sand Celebration!

1. Take a few long, deep cleansing breaths, with your eyes closed to block out any sensory messages.
2. Open your eyes.
3. Use the magickal energies of the deva's and elements you have connected to, through your bath; connect with Earth Mama as you inhale your sacred earth oils.
4. Take off your clothes (if possible and if you are comfortable).
5. Scan your body mentally.
6. Feel your body with your hands.
7. Spin and twirl, naturally, to get yourself in touch with the sacred spiral of the universe.
8. Translate and transcribe what you are feeling into words.
9. Write your words into the sand, erasing and writing more words, using your gather tools, as they come to you.

I can't see you right now, but words that come to mind for you, as a celebration for coming this far in your journey are:

Change	Joy	Acceptance
Beautiful	Wonder	

Feel free to borrow my words, which I'm sure are very appropriate for your state.

SKY CLAD

In several segments of paganism, Wicca and witchcraft, magick such as this affirmation ceremony, is done nude. Rather than being called nude or naked, it is called sky-clad. A word derived from Indian Religions' use of the word 'digambara', for monks that practice their spirituality without clothing. The word means sky-clad in English. If you can't practice sky-clad, as I suggest, please don a special ritual robe (I suggest white) or a lovely dress in your power color, scented with sandalwood, for this special occasion.

Completion Ritual

This book has been a journey into ways to engage the Earth Mama in your weight-loss journey. All the elements are important to her, and work that salutes her. So, before taking on your final day of ritual and ceremony, you will need to make, and request a few last things.

Play List (air/ether)

Ok, so this one is a snap. You will need a play list of your favorite songs or sounds to include in your celebratory ritual. What types of music inspire you?

- There are some great pagan albums, which invoke Earth Mama, various gods, goddesses and other spiritual beings.
- Some people like blues because they connect so deeply to dealing with adversity and struggle. Blues are also connected to the primal self and sexuality.
- Soul music, such as Aretha Franklin's "Respect," would make a nice addition.

- Earth sounds, such as storms (to stand for the storm you have weathered), rain for replenishment and renewal and crashing ocean waves, to connect to the healing power of water, and its beings, gods and goddesses.
- Use your imagination and cater to your personal taste.

Request Raw Food; Earthy Drink

Inform your circle of your intention for a closing celebration. Tell them that you've been following this book, and you are closing the circle it opened. Explain as much or as little as you wish about your journey to this point. Let them know, in the spirit of the work you have been doing, and the title of the book, "Earth Mama's Spiritual Guide to Weight-loss," you would like for them to bring simple, unadulterated food that comes directly from the earth. If it is a warm season, have them bring something from their garden or a local farmer's market. If it is colder their drinks could be centered around generating inner-warmth.

Ideas

Crudities	Herbal Tea (iced)
Fruit Salad	Mulled Wine
Vegetable Salad	Mead
Vegan Raw Food Recipes	Rum
Mixed Nuts	Sparkling Water

NOTE

Encourage the circle to treat this like a funeral reception, dressing accordingly in ritual robes or spiritual gear, and bringing flowers, if they would like.

The work:

Clay Figure (earth/water)

Supplies and Materials

You may purchase self-drying clay from any arts and crafts store.

You'll need a few sculpting tools for clay such as a wire cutting tool, a wooden pick tool and raking tool for texture.

Directions

- Create a large ball out of the clay that fits into your hand.
- Roll it out, gently and not super-thin.
- Sculpt your 'before-self', adding clay and subtracting clay where you see fit, until you have a representation of yourself that feels accurate.
- This can be abstract or representational. (No special art training needed and no judging allowed!)

Casket

Materials

A well-fitted bio-degradable box (shoe box, paint brush box, tea box, etc.,)

(Optional)

Burial objects (sample of addictive foods, sugar, notes, amulets, stones, or whatever you wish)

Paints, yarn, glitter glue, markers

Directions

Put burial objects you want to go with your 'before-self' under the ground, inside the casket.

Decorate the outside of the casket in any way you see fit, or leave it plain.

A Wake or Woke?

After someone has passed, many hold wakes. This is a gathering, often with food, which can now be used to tell stories – tales of remembrance, to grieve as a group, and to think of the future without that person, who was a part of your life. Once upon a time, wakes were to make sure the person was actually dead, and if their spirit appeared the family and friends were there to bear witness. Most of all, it is designed for safe passage.

In your case, you're not just at a-wake, you're woke! You have engaged with many types of spirituality and spiritual beings, hit (some of) your goals, worked out a strategy for maintaining them.

Procession and Burial

Ideally, you will have access to a space outdoors where you can bury your 'before-self'. Head to a sacred grove, forest or forest preserve; the sea (lake or pond), your yard or sacred garden. (If you do not have access to any of these natural spaces, use a soil-filled deep flower pot made for an indoor tree).

As you place your figure into the decorated or plain box, say:

You served me well old friend
Now it is time for you to be released from whence you came
Back to Earth Mama;
Repeat three times.

Have a couple of those in your circle carry the casket to the earth, where it will be buried.

Encourage the others in the group to clap and dancing the entire way, chanting: Back to Earth Mama You Go!

- Using a shovel dig an appropriate hole.
- Bury the casket with your figure inside.
- Leave a mound, so you know where your figure is buried.
- Pour a libation to guarantee safe passage to the land of your ancestors.
- Place the first flower on the mound; invite your guests to do the same.

Reception Celebration!

Now, it is time to Celebrate with your coven/healing circle (or friends and family) with libations, music, wholesome food, spirits and spontaneous song!

FINAL REFLECTIONS

When I started this book I wanted to:

_____

_____

_____

Now that I'm finished reading I intend to:

_____

The practice, god, goddess, being, lwa, orisha I want to learn more about to help with my weight-loss journey is:

_____

The altars I am intending to build are to whom and why?

_____

_____

_____

The altars I am tending are set for whom and why?

_____

_____

_____

Tomorrow is a very important day in this journey. What three things do you plan to do that utilizes the lessons of this book? Write them in order of importance!

1. _____

2. _____

3. _____

Continue your journey and to journal about your feelings along the way.

Congratulations and best of luck as you continue to work on the goals that mean the most to you!

Acknowledgements

Thank you first and foremost to Mama Earth, for inspiration, nurturing and support without end. A huge gratitude to Peter Gotto and the team at Green Magic Publishing, for believing in this project and supporting it throughout the publication process. Thank you to my husband, Damian for being my sounding board and partner in crime. Big, heartfelt thanks to my children for their boundless support, Ian, Olivia, Liam and Colin, and my soon-to-be son-in-law Xeno. To my British Mum and Dad, thank you for attentive listening and loving support, during my writing process. A special thank you to Lorin, my sister-in-law, for being supportive as I wrote, and to Julie and Susan, Jon and Ade, Samuel and Jaz for inspirational conversations by the seaside, and lending much needed support. Thanks also to my brothers, Mike and Rod for being patient, when I was too busy writing to talk, and my dear sister Rene, thank you also for your support. Jan, all those breakfast chats, coffees and lunches where we talked things out, have come to fruition – thank you for caring and for listening. Chun Hui, your willingness to be supportive and your actions speak louder than these words, a huge debt of gratitude. To my parents, relatives and ancestors who passed on and relatives scattered across the country, I always feel you are with me and know you are the wind at my back, propelling me forward.

Thank you all! To others I haven't mentioned but have felt your love, kindness and support along the way, I couldn't have done this without you.

Lightning Source UK Ltd.
Milton Keynes UK
UKOW05f0309030617

302609UK00002B/153/P

9 780995 547841